Spiritual Secrets to Weight Loss

Finally, a Permanent Solution

KARA DAVIS, M.D.

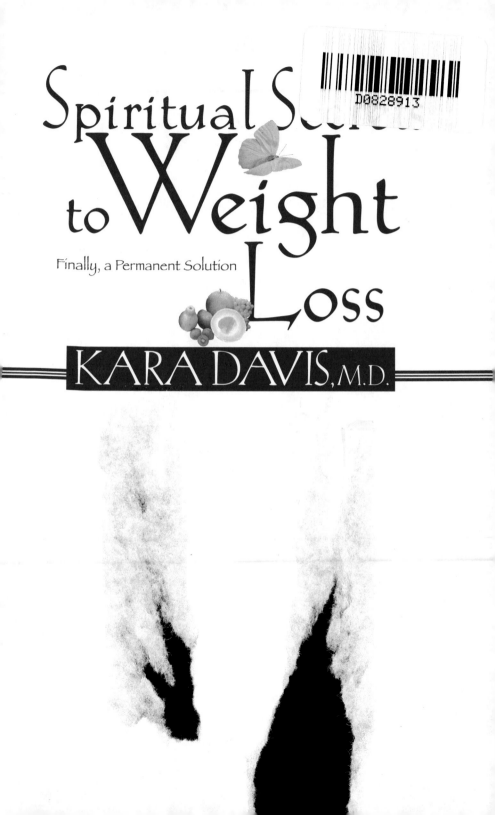

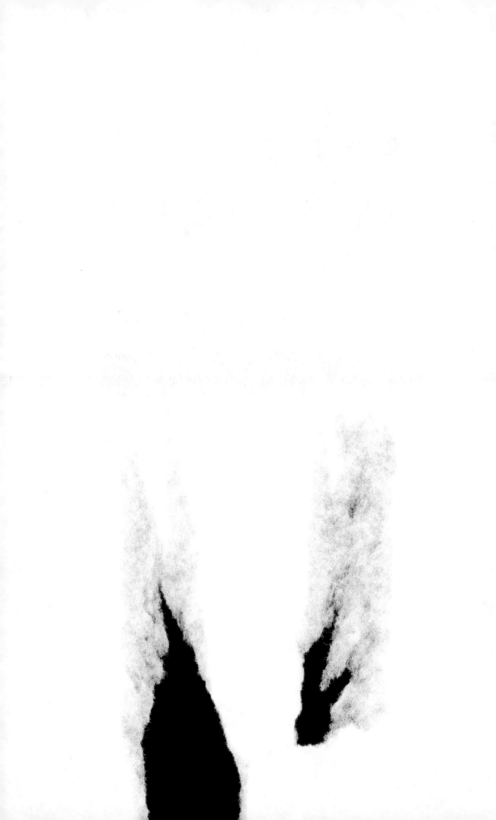

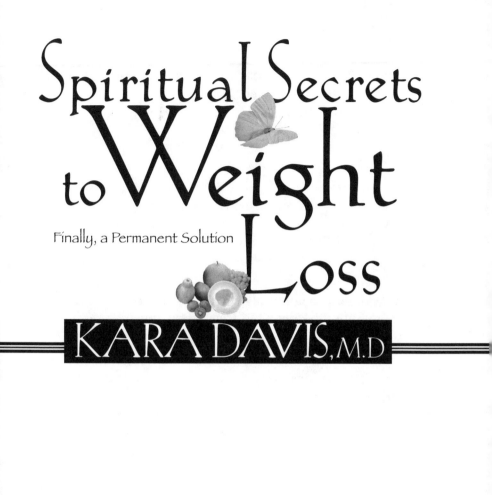

Spiritual Secrets
to Weight
Loss

Finally, a Permanent Solution

KARA DAVIS, M.D

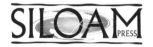

SILOAM PRESS

SPIRITUAL SECRETS OF WEIGHT LOSS by Kara E. Davis, M.D.
Published by Siloam Press
A part of Strang Communications Company
600 Rinehart Road
Lake Mary, Florida 32746
www.siloampress.com

Unless otherwise noted, all Scripture quotations marked
NIV are from the Holy Bible, New International Version.
Copyright © 1973, 1978, 1984, International Bible Society.
Used by permission.

Scripture quotations marked AMP are from the Amplified
Bible. Old Testament copyright © 1965, 1987 by the
Zondervan Corporation. The Amplified New Testament
copyright © 1954, 1958, 1987 by the Lockman Foundation.
Used by permission.

Scripture quotations marked KJV are from the
King James Version of the Bible.

Cover design by Karen Gonsalves

Library of Congress Catalog Card Number: 2002105201
International Standard Book Number: 0-88419-888-X

02 03 04 05 87654321
Printed in the United States of America

To my husband, pastor and best friend, Lance Davis, who stirred up the gift that was in me.

Contents

Introduction

Let the wise listen and add to their learning, and let the discerning get guidance.

—PROVERBS 1:5

But Dr. Davis, I don't eat that much! Will you check and see if there's a problem with my thyroid gland? How can I weigh more today than last month? Your scale must be wrong."

Sound familiar? Over the years, I have listened to a litany of complaints from my patients who struggle to lose weight. Their dieting efforts have a predictable outcome: Either they don't lose any weight at all, or they lose a few pounds only to gain them right back, sometimes ending up heavier than when they started. I see them in my office and share their frustration; their efforts, though seemingly valiant, availed nothing. Determination and sheer resolve seem to matter little in the weight loss arena.

I reiterate for them the connection between body weight and disease, and remind them that type 2 diabetes, hypertension, high cholesterol, arthritis and heart disease (to name but a few) are all exacerbated by obesity. Then we decide upon the lesser of two evils: Either I increase the dose of their current medications, or I prescribe yet another drug to add to their armamentarium of pills. I conclude our session by reviewing the pearls of wisdom they know so well: Don't eat before bedtime; read the food labels; use the stairs instead of the elevator; and bake, broil and boil, but never, ever, fry. It's the standard advice that they've already heard, if not from me, then from friends, on talk shows and in books and magazines. When it comes to weight loss, my patients usually have more helpful hints than I do. So why can't they lose weight?

This question vexed me. It was even more disturbing when I considered the subset of overweight people I treated in my office. These are people who have health problems that are directly related to their weight. While some overweight people are motivated to lose inches for purely cosmetic reasons, and others want to shed a few pounds in order to maintain their good health, my patients were physically ill, and they suffered from diseases that were caused by, or exacerbated by, their excessive weight. Sure, they wanted to feel comfortable wearing a bathing suit or shorts in the summer, but their main objective was to improve their health. They wanted to live long, healthy lives, but instead they were digging their own graves—one forkful at a time.

When it comes to weight loss, my patients usually have more helpful hints than I do. So why can't they lose weight?

My experience isn't unique, but it is one that is faced by healthcare professionals across the United States.

Over the past decade, there has been a steady increase in the prevalence of obesity in every state and across all age groups, races and educational levels. Statistics confirm that obesity is spreading "with the speed and dispersion characteristic of a communicable disease epidemic."[1]

All physicians, from the pediatrician to the geriatrician, are faced with this public health crisis. My patients and I were losing the battle; it seemed there was nothing we could do to succeed.

Nothing, that is, until I studied the problem from a different perspective. When I turned my attention away from the physical manifestations of obesity and focused instead on the spiritual needs of my patients, I realized then that their obesity was an indicator of an underlying spiritual problem. And since the battle was spiritual, weapons like will power and sheer determination were pretty ineffective. Likewise, doling out tips on diet and exercise rarely accomplished much.

> *I realized that their obesity was an indicator of an underlying spiritual problem.*

SPIRITUAL SECRETS

So I prayed for wisdom. As I prayed and studied the Bible, I discovered some wonderful answers provided for us there that I felt could help my patients. Of course, underlying spiritual problems cannot be resolved by our own efforts, will power or good intentions. They require the grace of God to change us through the power of the Holy Spirit as we learn to yield to Him. The commands of the Scriptures were never meant to be fulfilled in us by the efforts of the flesh. But they are meant to be fulfilled—by the wonderful grace that God gives to willing hearts that choose to obey. That obedience brings freedom from spiritual bondages of all kinds. The apostle Paul understood this when he wrote:

> So I say, live by the Spirit, and you will not gratify the desires of the sinful nature. For the sinful nature desires what is contrary to the Spirit, and the Spirit what is contrary to the sinful nature. They are in conflict with each other, so that you do not do what you want. But if you are led by the Spirit, you are not under law.
> —GALATIANS 5:16–18

Again, living by the Spirit is not something we can do in our own strength, as Paul explains. But as we learn to yield to the Holy Spirit within us, He empowers us to live in freedom from all bondage to our sinful nature. After listing some of the acts of our sinful nature, Paul contrasts them with the life in the Spirit:

> But the fruit of the Spirit is love, joy, peace, patience, kindness, goodness, faithfulness, gentleness and self-control. Against such things there is no law.
> —GALATIANS 5:22–23

When we allow the Holy Spirit to take control of our lives, these nine fruit of the Spirit begin to grow, displacing our sinful nature. These wonderful characteristics of divine life God has provided for us give us power to overcome the spiritual issues that lead to obesity. Cultivating them in our lives equips us to win the war on weight.

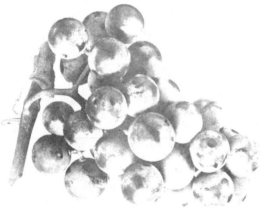

The commands of the Scriptures were never meant to be fulfilled in us by the efforts of the flesh.

As you learn to yield to the Holy Spirit, He will reveal the spiritual secrets that will enable you to conquer the roots of obesity in your life. My prayer is that as you read this book, the Lord will reveal to you those things you need to allow the Holy Spirit to change your life in order to experience victoriously good health.

Enjoy the fruit!

—KARA E. DAVIS, M.D.

One

The Fruit of the Spirit Is *Love . . .*

Hatred stirs up dissension, but love covers over all wrongs.
—PROVERBS 10:12

I f I made a list of personal grievances I have with the English language, the many uses (and abuses) of the word *love* would be close to the top of the list. Why is it that the same word that describes the profoundly intimate feeling a mother has for her child seems just as appropriate to use when describing our feeling for a piece of furniture, a style of clothing or even a place, like New York City? A clarification of terms is necessary for us to grasp the significance of love as defined for us by God.

LOVE IS . . .

The Greek language from which the New Testament was translated uses several different words to describe love. These words were applied appropriately for the conditions of love to which they referred.

Agape

For example, the Greek word *agape* describes love that is unconditional—*agape* is the essence of the Christian faith. It was this *agape* love of God for man that motivated Him to sacrifice His Son to restore His relationship with us: "For God so loved the world that he gave his one and only Son, that whoever believes in him shall not perish but have eternal life" (John 3:16).

Because of its divine origin, the term *agape* best describes the fruit of the Spirit of love. *Agape* love fulfills God's commandment to love our neighbors as ourselves (Matt. 19:19). It seeks the highest good for the recipient, even if he or she seems unworthy or even unappealing.

Agape is the love involving choice; we love unconditionally because we *will* to love. *Agape* love is not governed by our natural inclinations. It must at times ignore our natural emotional responses, choosing to love in spite of them. This is the love that covers all wrongs (Prov. 10:12).

Phileo

The Greek word for the "touchy-feely" kind of love is *phileo*. It refers to tender affection, that warmth and compassion we have toward the object of our love. The feeling experienced between good friends is typical *phileo* love. The recipient makes the giver feel good. This positive feedback is then the driving force that generates more *phileo* love.

Though *agape* and *phileo* love can coexist, we need to understand their essential differences. A healthy marriage or a normal parent-child relationship should manifest both *agape* love and *phileo* love. There should be an unconditional acceptance that covers wrongs in the relationships along with the "touchy-feely" response of *phileo*.

Unfortunately, it is *phileo* love that usually defines

love for us. This fact has been a source of confusion, especially among new believers, when they learn that as Christians we are commanded to love our enemies (Matt. 5:44). That seems difficult (if not impossible) to do if we are relating to the "touchy-feely" conditions of *phileo* love. How can we love an enemy the way we love a relative or a close friend? How can we feel *phileo* love—tenderness, warmth and affection—toward a person who has violated us and become our enemy?

Jesus never commanded us to love with *phileo* love. Instead, He asks that we love our enemies with *agape* love—the love that is based on a choice, not a feeling; the love that transcends the undesirable traits of the recipient; love that is unconditional. Of course, as we have mentioned, the source of *agape* love is God. He came to give His love to us and make it possible for us to experience unconditional love—for ourselves and others.

LOVING OURSELVES

When a man came to Jesus and asked how to receive eternal life, Jesus responded, "Do not murder, do not commit adultery, do not steal, do not give false testimony, honor your father and mother, and love your neighbor as yourself" (Matt. 19:18–19). It is rightly inferred from these commands that we must properly love ourselves, which in turn teaches us how to love our neighbor. And the word Jesus used for *love* in this command is *agape*—unconditional love based on choice.

Cultivating love for yourself is the first secret to becoming successful in the weight loss process. This may sound difficult because our society idolizes the thin physique and rejects the overweight. Obese people are subjected to discrimination in school, in the workplace and even among family. They are often labeled with negative stereotypes such as laziness, stupidity and poor hygiene. It should not be surprising that overweight people succumb to self-hatred as a reaction to society's perceived values. And the sting of that self-hatred is often assuaged through trips to the refrigerator—a strategy that only serves to exacerbate the problem.

In order to be successful in weight loss, we need to embrace the powerful secret of loving ourselves. That is why understanding the distinction between *agape* and *phileo* love is important. Choosing to love ourselves as God loves us, regardless of our physical appearance, is a correct application of *agape* love. It is a choice; it is unconditional; it is a biblical command.

In contrast, *phileo* self-love is unhealthy. It is at the root of such vices as haughtiness, selfishness and narcissism. *Agape* self-love reflects the acceptance God gives, unconditionally, of our person. We are created in the image of God, and according to the Scriptures, God is love (1 John 4:8). It is logical then, since we are created in the image of God, who loves us unconditionally, that we should love ourselves. Also, it impossible to fulfill Christ's command to love our neighbor as ourselves in the absence of godly self-love.

We have defined *agape* love as unconditional love motivated by choice. It is not swayed by the standards set by society; it does not require that we be satisfied with our physical condition or pleased with our appearance. When we love ourselves with *agape* love, we choose to seek the highest good for our spirit, mind and body, the recipients of that love, regardless of the way we feel about our bodies.

Success in weight loss requires lifestyle changes—changes that are always beneficial but quite often dramatic. The motivation that we need to implement these changes and the determination needed to stick with them require an unconditional love for the one who stands to benefit from the change. This is what *agape* self-love is all about. It empowers us to do what is best for our body, contrary to what our feelings may dictate.

As we mentioned, it is the work of the Holy Spirit to empower us to love ourselves properly, embracing this divine secret to weight loss. The apostle Paul told the believers at Corinth, "Do you not know that your body is a temple of the Holy Spirit, who is in you, whom you have received from God?" (1 Cor. 6:19). A temple is a sacred place that houses the presence of God.

> *It is the work of the Holy Spirit to empower us to love ourselves properly.*

Paul would have been quite familiar with temples, especially Solomon's temple built centuries before he wrote these words. He was also familiar with the words of the prophet Joel, who predicted that one day the Spirit of God would be poured out on all people. As Joel's prophecy is fulfilled in the hearts of believers and the Holy Spirit fills their lives, the temple of God is transformed from an inanimate structure to a living one—our spirit, mind and body. In Christ, we are the living temples of God. Self-love requires that we honor and respect the living temple. We can better understand this concept when we appreciate the significance of Solomon's temple.

THE TEMPLE OF GOD

The temple of God built by Solomon was well loved because that was where the people experienced the holy presence of God. Construction of this magnificent temple began in 952 B.C. and lasted for seven years. The materials and workmanship that went into the construction of Solomon's temple reinforce the significance of its value to the people. The construction site was sanctified as holy ground even before the first brick was laid. According to 1 Kings 6:7, "only blocks dressed at the quarry were used, and no hammer, chisel or any other iron tool was heard at the temple site while it was being built." We can't help but appreciate the awe and reverential fear that the people held regarding the Lord's dwelling place.

There are at least three valuable parallels between this inanimate structure and our bodies, the living temples of God, that relate to weight loss. Solomon's temple, along with our temples:

- Reflects parental involvement.

- Requires adequate maintenance.

- Restricts legitimate access.

As we discuss these important ideas, the Holy Spirit can begin to unlock the secrets to their success in our minds and hearts, preparing our temples to receive a fresh revelation of God's glory.

Reflects parental involvement

The inception of Solomon's temple began in his father's heart long before Solomon became king. King David, Solomon's father, wanted to build the temple himself, but God told him that his son would be the one to construct it. God would only allow David to gather materials and make preparation to build a temple. So while the actual construction took place under Solomon's rule, the preparations necessary to the building began out of the desire in his father's heart to construct a temple for God.

David purchased the land where the temple would be built long before the groundbreaking took place. He provided the "start-up capital" from his personal treasure amounting to 110 tons of gold and 260 tons of silver. He set aside the iron, stone and cedar logs necessary for construction, and he appointed stonecutters, masons and carpenters to work in its construction.

As a parent, David taught Solomon that God deserved a magnificent temple where He could be worshiped in a more real way than just receiving "lip service." Of course, David taught his son the importance of studying and obeying the precepts of God, but he also instilled in him a desire to honor God in a tangible way. Through David's example, Solomon learned that God's temple ought to reflect the worthiness of God. It was the dwelling place of El-Shaddai, God Almighty, and He deserved nothing less than the very best.

Our bodies, God's living temples, should be considered of utmost value as well—a home for the presence of God. But, unlike David, many parents today have not valued their own temples, and as a result, they are not instilling into their children the concept of valuing their bodies as a temple of God. They are not using sound wisdom and discretion in deciding what their children will eat, but permit them to fill up on junk foods that have little or no nutritional value.

This sad fact is evidenced by the national health crisis of childhood obesity. The most recent data suggest that 22 percent of children and adolescents are overweight, and 11 percent are obese, making obesity the most common health problem facing children.[1]

While obesity is affecting all children, those with obese parents are at a particularly high risk for becoming obese themselves. Certainly genetics plays a role, but we can't ignore the impact of the home environment through the parents' involvement in the child's health and the example set by the parents. David, through example and personal involvement, taught Solomon to place utmost value on building the temple of God. Parents today can teach their children, through example as well as their personal involvement, the value of their "living temples."

Loving the living temple. One of the more tangible ways to love our young living temples is to nourish their health through proper diet and exercise. In general, a parent controls most of the child's diet because the parent purchases and prepares the food. We can influence our children in their likes and dislikes of food by making the right kinds of foods available to them. For example, the current recommendations for children and adults are that we reduce the consumption of high-fat foods and increase the consumption of fruits and vegetables to five servings per day.

But in a study of close to two thousand elementary school children, 40 percent of them ate no vegetables on the days that the study was conducted, and 36 percent ate at least four different types of snack foods on the days they were studied—foods that tend to be high in fat.[2]

An even more recent study found that 80 percent of children and adolescents did not eat five or more servings of fruits and vegetables per day, but when a vegetable was eaten, 25 percent of the time it was French fries.[3]

At the same time, physical activity among children continues to decline. This too results from a lack of parental involvement. Parents have allowed many public school systems to reduce the amount of time devoted to physical education. In some cases, the physical education class is sedentary because it's used for courses like health and driver's education. Parents have allowed outdoor playtime to be replaced with television and video games. And they are more willing to drive children to places close enough to walk. Most importantly, parents are not engaging in regular exercise themselves. They are setting the unhealthy example of how to become a "couch potato."

Parents are responsible for bringing the obesity epidemic of children under control. They must teach their children the importance of maintaining good health through proper diet and exercise. Their instruction will have more influence if they can reinforce it through example. Exercising with your children could open avenues for relationship that would be positive in every way. Children should see their parents choosing a healthy lifestyle and know that they are motivated by a love for God and a desire to properly care for His living temple.

Requires adequate maintenance

Thirty-eight thousand Levitical priests were responsible for the upkeep of Solomon's temple: Twenty-four thousand supervised temple activities, six thousand served as judges and officials, four thousand were gatekeepers, and four thousand were musicians. They worked in shifts throughout the year and were supported financially by the nation of Israel, even during the times that they weren't on duty. The temple received this kind of adequate maintenance because it was valued as the dwelling place of God.

But what happens to our living temples? Along with subjecting ourselves to excess stress and inadequate rest (which would be bad enough), we also fail to provide ourselves with a nutritious diet and sufficient exercise. It is a fact that diets that are nutritionally depleted will lack the vitamins and minerals necessary to protect us against diseases such as cancer and coronary artery disease. And the combination of a poor diet and a lack of exercise will lead to weight gain and all the medical problems associated with being overweight.

Many people are falling short in the area of temple maintenance. Understanding *agape* love—loving by choice—will help us make right choices to become motivated to implement a healthy lifestyle. As we grow in our love for God, we will desire to nurture His dwelling place, our bodies. As we choose to love ourselves, we will be freed from the bondages to habits that caused destruction in our temples.

Restricts legitimate access

Animal sacrifice took place every day in Solomon's temple, but there were restrictions placed on which species were acceptable to God. According to Mosaic Law, sacrificial animals had to be "clean." Animals with an incompletely divided split hoof (like pigs) or animals that moved around close to the ground (like rats or weasels) were deemed "unclean"; they were not eaten and were unacceptable for sacrifice.

This concept of restricting access also applies to our living temples. Not everything that is touted as edible should find access to our living temples. Some theologians contend that New Testament doctrine has removed the dietary restrictions of the Mosaic Law. Even if that is true, it does not remove the need to use discretion and constraint when it comes to what we eat.

There are certain diseases, like type 2 diabetes, high cholesterol and hypertension, for which diet modification is the first line of therapy. Medications are considered second-line therapy—they do not replace the need to modify the diet, but are used when diet alone is ineffective. Many people with these conditions are able to control them without medications; they simply adhere to the prescribed diet that is proper for maintaining health. But an alarming number choose to disregard these dietary recommendations. Foods that should be eaten on rare occasions become part of the regular menu.

Because they fail to abide by the principle of restricted access, they suffer the consequences of these diseases, consequences that are always serious and sometimes even life threatening. One of the benefits of *agape* love is that it motivates us to set restrictions on the types of food we eat and learn to control the amount we consume. Food should edify and fortify our bodies, not destroy them. We should apply a greater intensity of tender loving care to our living temple than that which was given to Solomon's temple, an inanimate structure.

SACRIFICIAL LOVE

Every time I'm in the supermarket checkout line, I see a tabloid or magazine featuring a diet plan that allows you to eat as much as you like, of whatever you like. These miracle diets promise radical weight loss in the absence of radical lifestyle changes. It seems as if a new plan is created each week, attesting to our tendency to want something for nothing. We like to have our cake, eat it too and shed a few pounds in the process.

Even though what these diet plans promise defies logic, we are willing to forsake our common sense and give them a chance. I was once told that if something seemed too good to be true, it probably was. This truth applies to these dime-a-dozen weight loss schemes. They simply don't work in either the short term or, more importantly, in the long run.

So why, then, do we feel compelled to try them? We have not understood a key aspect of love: Love requires sacrifice. Love, fully expressed, will usually require that we relinquish something of value.

It is interesting that most of the items acceptable for Old Testament sacrifices were edible: grain, oil, wine and meat. The animals offered were livestock that would have otherwise been used for food, not beasts of burden like mules and donkeys. An animal needed to meet two criteria in order to be an acceptable sacrifice. First, the item offered had to be without blemish, and second, it had to be owned by the one relinquishing it.

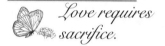

Love requires sacrifice.

Offer the best. In the Book of Malachi, God issues this rebuke to the people for their failure to offer Him their best:

> "When you bring injured, crippled or diseased animals and offer them as sacrifices, should I accept them from your hands?" says the LORD. "Cursed is the cheat who has an acceptable male in his flock and vows to give it, but then sacrifices a blemished animal to the Lord. For I am a great king," says the LORD Almighty, "and my name is to be feared among the nations."
> —MALACHI 1:13–14

After the acceptable animal was slaughtered, its blood was sprinkled on the altar and its body divided. The purpose of the sacrifice would determine whether the entire animal or just parts of the animal were burned. In some cases, the unburned remains were given to the priest; at other times, the person presenting the offering took the remains home to eat. But in all cases, the choice parts of the animal—the entrails and the fat—were completely burned to provide "an aroma pleasing to the LORD" (Lev. 1:9).

An unacceptable sacrifice. The Bible records the sacrifice of two brothers, Cain and Abel, and God's response to each one. (See Genesis 4.) Abel brought a sacrifice of the firstlings of his flock, their fat portions. Cain, his brother, brought to the Lord an offering of the fruit of the ground. Cain's offering was rejected by God, and the anger that ensued led him to murder Abel.

While the Bible does not explicitly state why God responded as He did to these brothers' sacrifices, commentators agree that the sovereign God would have had a good reason to reject one and accept the other. The Bible says that Abel selected the finest he had to offer—the "fat portions from some of the firstborn of his flock" (Gen. 4:4). But the description of Cain's offering says only that he "brought some of the fruits of the soil as an offering to the Lord" (v. 3)—there is no indication that he carefully chose the pick of the crop. It seems that God was not pleased with the quality of the sacrifice Cain brought and with the attitude in which it was offered.

Ownership required. The second criterion for an acceptable sacrifice was that the item relinquished be owned by the individual making the offering. This Old Testament system of worship required that a food item be relinquished by the owner with the understanding that if any part of it was to be returned and eaten, it would be a smaller portion and would not include the parts highest in fat. A person did not sacrifice in his own behalf something that belonged to someone else.

We know, for example, that King David purchased the land for the temple that was eventually built by his son Solomon. Araunah, owner of the land, offered to give it to David free of charge. And as king, David could have confiscated the land (whether Araunah offered it or not), or at least paid an amount far less than the land's value. But David told Araunah, "No, I insist on paying you for it. I will not sacrifice to the LORD my God burnt offerings that cost me nothing" (2 Sam. 24:24). The king knew that an offering without ownership was meaningless; he paid the full price.

Purpose for sacrifice

The act of sacrifice required a person to give up something of value that belonged to him. The Jewish people knew they were to continue this sacrificial system all their life; their worship of God required it. But why did God ordain this practice? Certainly, God did not "need" the sacrifice; the person presenting the offering was doing God no favor. What, then, was the purpose?

It was simply a way to tangibly express thankfulness to God for His goodness and His mercy, providing restitution as well for any offense committed against God. In other words, it was a way to express love. This sacrificial ritual, which was part of their worship of God, was performed daily; it was a regular part of Jewish life, not a seasonal or holiday activity. Two lambs, a grain offering, olive oil and wine were part of the daily offering. A more elaborate offering was presented on the Sabbath to show their love for God.

From the start, the practice was subject to corruption

because of religious hypocrites who turned it into a pointless ritual. But despite this tendency toward corruption, the Bible records for us lives of individuals who offered sincere and meaningful sacrifices of love that pleased God.

For example, God asked Abraham to sacrifice Isaac, his son. (See Genesis 22.) Abraham cherished Isaac; he was the long-awaited child promised to him by God. Yet, his willingness to sacrifice his son was proof of Abraham's unwavering faith, his obedience and, most importantly, his love for the Lord. Who can read God's poignant response to Abraham's obedience without sensing the depth of love it reveals: "Now I know that you fear God, because you have not withheld from me your son, your only son"(Gen. 22:12).

Sacrifice is not exclusive to the Old Testament. Paul, in his epistle to the Romans, wrote, "Therefore, I urge you, brothers, in view of God's mercy, to offer your bodies as living sacrifices, holy and pleasing to God— this is your spiritual act of worship" (Rom. 12:1). Sacrifice is still required, but our offering is no longer the best pick of our crop or the nicest lamb in our flock. Instead, we symbolically place ourselves—our very own bodies—on the altar of the Lord. We are living sacrifices; we lay aside our own desires to embrace a higher purpose—our love for God.

If we love God, then we must express that love toward His temple, our bodies. We do that when we make a commitment to live a healthy lifestyle, even if it requires us to "sacrifice" something we enjoy. The tabloid diets have such an appeal because they promise the "gain" of weight loss without the "pain" of sacrifice. But the old adage is true: no pain, no gain. Permanent weight loss only happens when there is a willingness to embrace sacrifice as a vital part of love.

A positive approach. Changing our behavior to improve our health is a positive choice, even though it involves sacrifice. We need to overcome the tendency to view sacrifice in a negative light. Sacrifice is not penance, nor is it a form of torture. It should not be done begrudgingly, but with an attitude of joyful thanksgiving. Sacrifice is a manifestation of love, and our attitude toward a healthful lifestyle should reflect that love.

The average person thinks of a "diet" in terms of temporary deprivation, not a lifestyle change. The result of that kind of thinking is a *goal-oriented* mind-set. The primary focus then becomes the "end" of the diet, whether that happens to be next week, next month or even next year. We promise ourselves, *If I can continue with this agony for just a little longer, I'll be able to fit into that dress.* Our temporary deprivation has a goal to meet a specified end.

The worst part about this attitude is that along with anticipation of the end, there is also a plan for rewarding ourselves upon reaching the goal, usually with the very foods that were temporarily denied. From day one, we start to think about those reward foods—the cheesecake and the ice cream—that will be eaten with abandon once the goal is met. We set ourselves up to fail, regaining whatever weight was lost. And we pervert the true purpose of food as nourishment. Instead of being neutral, it takes on a life of "good" or "bad," a "reward" or a "punishment."

In order to succeed at losing weight—permanently—we must stop thinking in terms of temporary change. We don't need a "diet" that changes our menu for a week or two; we need a "diet" that will permanently change our attitude about food, our health and the way we treat God's living temple. Our attitude must reflect a spirit of sacrificial love, which makes us willing to give up a few things we enjoy for the greater purpose of good health.

> *We need a "diet" that will permanently change our attitude about food, our health and the way we treat God's living temple.*

Over the years, those patients in my practice who have been successful at losing weight have all come to terms with the inevitability of sacrifice. Their testimonies are never affirmations that losing weight was an easy thing to do. Instead, they confirm that success was dependent upon changing a behavior or eliminating a habit:

- ❧ "I started cooking more beans and lentils, and now I eat less meat."

- ❧ "I used to buy a candy bar on my way home from work, but I stopped doing that."

- ❧ "Now I get out of bed a half-hour earlier to exercise on my treadmill."

It's all about sacrifice—a willingness to forgo something we might enjoy (whether meat, sweets or an extra half-hour of sleep) for the higher purpose of good health. Making the sacrifice will be more difficult for some than for others. If food is used to nurture the emotions, or if it has a strong psychological significance, then making the sacrifice will be difficult.

In that case, the first step is to come to terms with those problems that are being placated with food, which we will discuss further. Likewise, if the problem is not so much excessive eating as it is a lack of exercise, then the sacrifice will require a time commitment, which may not be easy for busy people. No matter what the situation, a sacrifice is required.

Some foods require a total sacrifice. Whole milk, for example, should be given up completely and replaced with reduced fat or skim milk because of its negative effects on our health. Other foods require a partial sacrifice. We don't have to totally eliminate them from our diet, but we should restrict them in terms of their serving size and frequency with which we eat them. For example, ice cream does not have to be completely eliminated, but it shouldn't be eaten every day by the pint. Butter is to be used in small amounts with moderation, not lavished on every item on the plate.

Weight loss only comes through the sacrifice of an unhealthy lifestyle. We have bought into the notion that losing weight should be easy, but this is simply not true. It requires sacrifice...

℘ Of unhealthy foods that we eat for comfort or psychological reasons

- ❧ Of time to devote to exercise

- ❧ Of other unhealthy habits that are currently part of our lifestyle

A *hard teaching*

Simply put, some foods and some eating habits must be placed on the altar and symbolically burned. They need to be sacrificed willingly out of love for God and a desire to do whatever it takes to keep His living temple free from disease and illness. What makes us willing to sacrifice a lifestyle that is comfortable to us? What allows us to maintain a new way of living?

Love (*agape* love) provides the strength we need to make the sacrifice. God fills us with His love, which empowers us to make whatever sacrifice is necessary to bring glory to Him in our temples. If you have not experienced this *agape* love, God is waiting to reveal Himself to you in a new way. He will teach you to love yourself as His temple, and He will empower you to do so.

The Gospel of John records that many of Jesus' disciples grumbled after hearing His revolutionary teaching. Jesus was teaching that He was the bread of life and that we must eat that bread to live forever (John 6:51). They said to each other, "This is a hard teaching. Who can accept it?" (v. 60). Some did not accept it; they turned away and no longer followed him. Their turning away did not change the validity of Jesus' teachings; it only demonstrated that even some who followed Jesus were not ready to accept the truth.

The need for sacrifice is also a hard teaching, and not everyone will be able to accept it. The promoters of fad diets and weight loss schemes have convinced us that losing weight should be easy and effortless. They have so persuaded us that any suggestion to the contrary is not readily accepted. However, all we need to do is take a look around us to see that one out of every three or four people is overweight or obese. This observation alone ought to make us suspicious of the weight loss industry's claims. If losing weight is as easy as they claim, where are the results they promise?

Keep in mind that the weight loss business is quite lucrative. In 1996, Americans spent an estimated $35 billion in an effort to lose weight.[4]

When that kind of money is being doled out on an annual basis, be assured that many are going to try to get a piece of the "weight loss pie," and they will follow the old principle of supply and demand—give the people what they want. We want a simple and painless solution to a complex problem, so diets are created that are simple and pain free. It doesn't matter whether they work or not; what matters is that the capitalists have gotten their share of the billions.

The truth of the matter is that losing weight requires that we change our lifestyles, and change does not come easily. So how do we become motivated, and where do we find the power to implement such dramatic changes? If the Spirit of God is in us, we have the motivating force, the power source, with us all the time. Scripture teaches that "God has poured out his love into our hearts by the Holy Spirit" (Rom. 5:5). The fruit of the Spirit of love—*agape* love—will help us, first by adjusting our attitudes about our bodies. We are not merely bones and flesh, but we are the living temples of God, and, as such, we are of great value to God.

Once we embrace the wonderful truth that we are God's living temple, the fruit of the Spirit of love empowers us to make whatever sacrifices are required to keep our temples healthy. We will find the strength we need as we open our hearts to this spiritual secret—the power of love. As we grow in the fruit of the Spirit of love, sacrifice becomes easier because our deepest desire will be to love and please God.

TWO

The Fruit of the Spirit Is *Joy* . . .

A cheerful heart is good medicine, but a
crushed spirit dries up the bones.
—PROVERBS 17:22

It was not long after my husband became a pastor that we recognized the need for a separate children's service. The children were not unwelcome in the main service, but their boredom was obvious. Despite the activity bags that their parents filled with snacks, crayons and coloring books, they were fidgety and restless soon after the service began.

We felt that unless things changed, the children would dread Sunday. Church service would become a weekly test of their endurance, and once they were old enough, they would likely stop attending altogether. So we laid the foundation for our Children's Church. Our objective was to create a service where children could worship God at their own level and to make Sunday a day they eagerly anticipated.

Once our Children's Church was established, it didn't take long for the children to discover that worshiping the Lord was fun. They even began inviting their friends. They learned that God wanted everyone, even children, to rejoice in His presence with singing, dancing and celebration. We were able to teach them what many adults had long since forgotten—that one of the benefits of serving the Lord is experiencing His joy.

Throughout all of Scripture, we are admonished to rejoice and be glad. For Christians, joy is much more than a happy feeling. As a fruit of the Spirit, joy dwells within us at all times, independent of our circumstances.

Why, then, are so many Christians not experiencing the joy of the Spirit? Jesus promised that His joy would not only be present in His followers, but also that it would be complete and overflowing (John 15:11). Joy does not forsake the believer in whom the Holy Spirit dwells. It can, however, be suppressed. Suppression is an important factor in the cause of clinical depression.

DEPRESSION: THE JOY SNATCHER

There is much wisdom in the old adage that laughter is the best medicine. The scientific community is finally accepting what the Bible has taught all along—that there is a close connection between the mind and the body. A recent study published in the *Archives of Internal Medicine* found that, in older individuals, even mild levels of depression increased the risk of death from *any* cause. Those suffering with severe depression had a 35 percent higher risk of dying within six years than those with low levels of depression.[1]

Studies such as these confirm that our physical condition is tightly linked to our mental attitude. Stated differently, the state of our physical health is positively or negatively influenced by our state of mind. Scripture supports this scientific conclusion. The Book of Proverbs contains excellent advice about how to stay healthy by maintaining a positive mental attitude. Consider the following verses:

> A cheerful heart is good medicine, but a crushed spirit dries up the bones.
>
> —PROVERBS 17:22

> A happy heart makes the face cheerful, but heartache crushes the spirit.
>
> —PROVERBS 15:13

> A cheerful look brings joy to the heart, and good news gives health to the bones.
>
> —PROVERBS 15:30

> Pleasant words are a honeycomb, sweet to the soul and healing to the bones.
>
> —PROVERBS 16:24

> A man's spirit sustains him in sickness, but a crushed spirit who can bear?
>
> —PROVERBS 18:14

So the manifestations of joy—a happy heart, a cheerful countenance and pleasant words—have the power to protect our health, according to the Scriptures. And the "crushed spirit" of depression can cause, or exacerbate, physical illness.

NOT JUST A CASE OF "THE BLUES"

Every now and then, we all feel a little down and out. Life is often filled with trouble, and discouraging circumstances abound, so occasional feelings of sadness are quite normal. We may, like the psalmist, find ourselves asking, "Why are you downcast, O my soul?

Why so disturbed within me?" (Ps. 42:11). It is normal to have times when we feel "downcast" in the face of life's challenges.

Unfortunately, some people feel more than just an occasional bout with "the blues." For them, the feelings of depression are overwhelming and unexplained. They are consumed with a sense of sadness that has no identifiable source. In these instances, the symptoms cannot be attributed to those normal, transient periods of feeling down and out. Instead, they indicate a clinical depression.

The person suffering with depression may feel sad, helpless and irritable. Changes in sleeping patterns are also common, taking the form of insomnia, excessive sleep or restless sleep. In some cases, depression may distort the thought processes, even to the point of causing delusions and hallucinations. The appetite may be affected, resulting in either anorexia or overeating. Fatigue and a lack of interest in the activities once enjoyed are also symptoms of clinical depression. Job performance and school performance suffer because of an inability to concentrate. In severe cases, there are recurring thoughts of suicide and death.

Signs of depression can be elusive. It often goes undiagnosed because many people don't attribute their symptoms to depression. They think they have some other condition, like the flu or anemia. This explains why a great number of depressed people first seek help from a primary care physician—an internist or a family doctor—and not a psychiatrist. They believe their symptoms are the result of an organic, rather than a psychiatric, disorder.

Clinical depression is extremely common. In any given six-month period, approximately 9.4 million Americans suffer with it. It is estimated that one out of every four women, and one out of every ten men, will experience at least one bout of depression during their lifetime. Part of the gender discrepancy can be attributed to the increased incidence of depression in women of childbearing age. Over 10 percent of new mothers experience a major depression during the first year after giving birth. Postpartum depression is different from "maternity blues," which is a mild, self-limited "down in the dumps" disposition that some feel is a normal reaction to childbirth since it occurs in so many women—fully 50 to 80 percent of women have it during the first two weeks after delivery.[2]

Depression is also a major problem for the elderly. Nearly five million of the thirty-one million Americans over the age of sixty-five have significant depressive symptoms.[3]

Depression falls into the category of mental illnesses known as the *affective disorders*. I have included here the main symptoms of major and minor depression as listed by the American Psychiatric Association. Certain symptoms are more specific for depression than others. Thoughts of suicide, for instance, are very specific for depression, while other symptoms such as fatigue and insomnia are not as specific. Clinicians use the mnemonic (memory device) of "SPACE DIGS" to help establish the diagnosis and determine which depressive syndrome is appropriate for their patient. (There is a third depressive syndrome, *dysthymia*, which falls in intensity between major and minor depression).

SYMPTOMS AND DIAGNOSTIC CRITERIA FOR DEPRESSIVE DISORDERS

Less Depression-Specific Symptoms

S leep disturbance (either insomnia or hyper-somnia)

P sychomotor retardation or agitation

A ppetite disturbance (decreased or increased) or weight loss or gain

C oncentration difficulties

E nergy low (i.e., tiredness, fatigue)

More Depression-Specific Symptoms

D epressed mood

I nterest in normal activities is diminished or lost

G uilt or feelings of worthlessness—excessive or inappropriate

S uicidal ideation or thoughts of death

~~~

According to the American Psychiatric Association, you may be suffering from major depression if at least five of the listed symptoms have been present nearly every day for two or more weeks and at least one of the symptoms is depressed mood or diminished interest in normal activities. You may be suffering from minor depression (still considered a mood disorder) if two to four of the depressive symptoms have been present nearly every day for at least two weeks, and at least one of the symptoms is depressed mood or loss of interest in normal activities.

Some medical disorders left untreated (for example, hypothyroidism) can cause depression. Before diagnosing depression, a patient must be screened for these diseases. The diagnosis of depression is deferred when a person has an identifiable life stressor, such as the death of a loved one. The depressed mood is then attributed to a grief reaction—a normal response to adversity—rather than a clinical depression. Occasionally, however, the bereavement period is prolonged, or the symptoms of grief fail to ease with time. In these instances, the stressful event has triggered clinical depression.

People suffering depression are more likely to become physically ill than people who are not depressed. The converse is also true, that depression may worsen the prognosis for some medical conditions. A major study on cardiovascular disease showed that patients who suffered a heart attack and subsequently developed depression were more likely to die in the six months following their heart attack than those patients who had a heart attack but did not become depressed.[4] And even those heart disease patients who survive don't fare as well in the face of depression. A study published in 1999 found that middle-aged and older persons with coronary heart disease and high scores for depressive symptoms reported higher rates of physical disability than those patients with low scores.[5]

The association between depression and an unfavorable outcome in people with coronary heart disease has been confirmed in so many major studies that it is now fairly standard for cardiac rehabilitation programs to include some form of psychosocial therapy, along with physical therapy. One such study involved an analysis of a few thousand patients. The investigators uncovered an interesting finding: The 2,024 patients who received psychosocial treatment not only had greater reductions in psychosocial distress, but they also had lower blood pressures, heart rates and cholesterol levels than the 1,156 patients who did not receive psychosocial treatment. The untreated group was also noted to have a greater mortality rate and a higher likelihood of having additional heart problems during the two years that they were followed.[6] Depression also has a negative influence on diseases other than heart disease, including cancer, type 2 diabetes and, of course, obesity.

OBESITY AND DEPRESSION

Obesity and depression go hand in hand. It is estimated that about 25 to 30 percent of obese patients who seek weight reduction treatment suffer with a significant depression or other psychological disturbance.[7] Many of these patients have binge eating disorder, a fairly common eating disorder occurring in 2 percent of the general population, more commonly in women.

Binge eating disorder is similar to bulimia nervosa in that patients experience a loss of control while eating and consume large quantities of food at a single sitting. They eat to the point of being uncomfortably full, but unlike bulimics, binge eaters do not make themselves vomit, and they don't abuse laxatives. Depression is frequently diagnosed in binge eaters.

Since both obesity and depression are common conditions, it's often difficult to determine if one is related to the other or if the person afflicted with both conditions simply has two common problems, occurring simultaneously, but totally unrelated to one another. Statisticians refer to this as "association vs. causation."

When an obese person is also depressed, it helps to know if the obesity is merely associated with the depression or if there is a cause-and-effect relationship. If the answer is one of *causation*, rather than just *association*, then the depression must be addressed as part of the overall approach to weight loss.

Once it is determined that obesity and depression have a causative relationship, it's tempting to try and figure out which one is causing the other. The two conditions have a "chicken and egg" dynamic: Did the depression make the person obese, or did the obesity make the person depressed? But while it may be interesting to know the "source" condition, the answer is purely academic since the solution is the same—treat the depression.

Why is it that it's nearly impossible to succeed in losing weight in the face of untreated depression? Because eating behavior and the attitude toward exercise are both influenced by depression. Depression leads to overeating when food is used to soothe its symptoms. And depression destroys motivation, which is so necessary to prompt regular exercise.

To make matters worse, depression can be triggered by repeated failures with weight loss plans, an experience common to most people who have attempted to lose weight. The typical dieter will experiment with several weight loss plans that ultimately fail. The failure is usually apparent from the start: The dieter never loses any pounds despite adhering to the plan's instructions. More devastating, though, is the plan that starts off well but fails in the long run. In this instance, the dieter may lose a considerable amount of weight, but regain every pound over the course of weeks, months or even years.

So the dieter subjects himself to cycles of hope and despair, which are powerful triggers for depression. The initial hope that *this* will be the diet, *this* will be the program, *this* will be the plan that finally works is ultimately destroyed by failing to reach the goal. On the surface, the dieter might attribute failure to the plan itself, criticizing the manufacturer for making such outrageous claims. But on the inside, he holds himself responsible, shouldering the blame for attempting an unrealistic and impractical diet plan. When failure is internalized the end result is a damaged sense of self-worth: *Not only am I overweight; I am an overweight failure.*

If the dieter musters the courage to try again and experiments with another plan that ultimately fails, the cycle repeats itself, and the already damaged sense of self-worth falls another notch lower. Each unsuccessful attempt to lose weight reinforces this association between being overweight and being a failure. Continual discouragement and defeat lead to depression.

THE CAUSE, THE CURE

While it is clear that depression can be triggered by

events like the death of a loved one, divorce or the cycle of hope and despair so often experienced by the dieter, the actual *cause* of depression remains unknown. The scientific community cannot explain why some people become depressed when faced with adversity while others in similar circumstances do not. An even more perplexing observation is that severe depression will often afflict those who are living what appear to be perfect and carefree lives.

Although the cause is unclear, several factors are linked to the development of depression:

- ❧ Depression tends to run in families and is more common in women, which suggests a *genetic* predisposition.

- ❧ Social factors play a role. People who have secure and stable relationships are less likely to become depressed than those who do not. The divorced and separated have a twofold to fourfold increased risk of depression compared to married people.

- ❧ The significance of healthy relationships in protecting against depression is confirmed by international data, which shows a low incidence of depression in cultures where there are strong community and family ties.

- ❧ There is evidence that an imbalance in the levels of neurotransmitters contributes to the development of depression. Some of the more interesting data regarding the origin of depression relate to various chemicals in the brain, known as neurotransmitters. Several effective antidepressant medications work by changing the concentrations of these chemicals.

ح Grief following the death of a spouse often leads to depression. A third of those who lose a spouse have symptoms consistent with major depression in the first month after the death, and half of these remain depressed one year later.

ح Major illness increases the likelihood of depression. The depressive disorders are two to three times more common in nursing home residents, hospitalized patients and patients with chronic medical problems.

Drugs have been developed as one form of treatment for depression. One category of antidepressant drugs is known as the serotonin-reuptake inhibitors. They alter the brain's concentration of the neurotransmitter serotonin. Some of the drugs in this particular class were found to have an interesting side effect: They suppress the appetite. This gives credence to the theory that mood and eating behavior are linked. If we accept this theory, then it's easy to conclude that the best way to treat both depression and obesity is with medications. But even though medications may work well, they are not the only forms of therapy to consider. Behavioral therapy and psychotherapy—for groups or individuals—are also quite effective and do not require the use of drugs.

The issue is further complicated by the well-known

placebo effect. In a review of seventy-five clinical trials involving patients with major depressive disorder, the response to a placebo ranged from 10 to 50 percent. In about half of the trials, 30 percent or more of the patients who were taking a placebo showed a significant improvement in their depressive symptoms.[8] So even if the problem originates from a chemical imbalance, the solution to correcting the imbalance does not always require the use of prescription drugs. I personally believe that, for the Christian, the best form of therapy is a personal choice—to experience *joy*.

CHOOSE JOY

True joy can lift us out of the depths of depression and give us the power that we need to succeed in losing weight. What does joy look like? In the Bible, particularly in the Old Testament, joy denotes a feeling of exuberance and gladness. Joy was outwardly expressed through singing, shouting and dancing. For example, King David leaped and danced with joy when he returned the ark of the covenant to Jerusalem (2 Sam. 6:14). Psalm 100 begins with this exhortation: "Shout for joy to the LORD, all the earth. Worship the LORD with gladness; come before him with joyful songs" (vv. 1–2).

Joy and depression, like light and darkness, are contrary to one another.

But joy has an even deeper source than the emotions, and its expression extends beyond mere feelings of gladness. Joy, as a fruit of the Spirit, resides in the Christian; it is present at all times, regardless of negative circumstances. I have concluded, after much observation, that depression cannot prevail in the person who has a firm understanding of the fruit of the Spirit of joy.

Joy and depression, like light and darkness, are contrary to one another. As such, they cannot coexist. This is not to say that there are no depressed Christians—there are. But as Christians, when we recognize depression is working in us we can make use of the most effective form of therapy. Choosing to experience God's divine joy should be step one in the treatment plan.

It is important to understand that experiencing joy and feeling happy are not synonymous. Happiness, like the *phileo* love we discussed in the last chapter, is dependent upon circumstances. Joy, however, relates to *agape* love; it is unconditional. If the Spirit of God dwells in us (as He does all Christians), joy is present, even in times of sorrow and despair.

Experience teaches us that grief and disappointment are a part of life—they touch the lives of Christians and non-Christians alike. Jesus warned us of this fact. In John 16:33, He says, "In this world you will have trouble. But take heart! I have overcome the world." It is not normal to feel happy during times of trouble. But joy is different. When faced with adversity, and when the pain from trials and circumstances is severe, according to the Bible, we can still "take heart." In other words, our joy is not destroyed by any of the unhappy conditions of this world.

Experiencing joy does not exempt us from feeling pain. Even Jesus experienced intense sorrow. In the Garden of Gethsemane, He agonized to the point that He perspired blood (Luke 22:44). Joy does not remove the pain that comes from adversity, but it will influence the outcome in our souls. Grief takes one of two courses: It will either subside, or it will persist and lead to depression. Joy is able to steer the grieving process down the path toward resolution.

> *Our joy is not destroyed by any of the unhappy conditions of this world.*

Inspired by the apostle Paul

Paul became a Christian on the road to Damascus. His conversion experience temporarily blinded him, and God instructed a man named Ananias to lay hands on Paul in order to restore his sight. At first, Ananias resisted, but the Lord gave him some information about Paul's destiny:

> Go! This man is my chosen instrument to carry my name before the Gentiles and their kings and before the people of Israel. I will show him how much he must suffer for my name.
>
> —ACTS 9:15–16

From the start of Paul's ministry, God made it clear that he was ordained to suffer. And suffer he did. He summarized the many times he was persecuted for the sake of Christianity in a letter he wrote to the

Corinthian church for the purpose of validating his authority with the believers in that city:

> I have worked much harder, been in prison more frequently, been flogged more severely, and been exposed to death again and again. Five times I received from the Jews the forty lashes minus one. Three times I was beaten with rods, once I was stoned, three times I was shipwrecked, I spent a night and a day in the open sea, I have been constantly on the move. I have been in danger from rivers, in danger from bandits, in danger from my own countrymen, in danger from Gentiles; in danger in the city, in danger in the country, in danger at sea; and in danger from false brothers. I have labored and toiled and have often gone without sleep; I have known hunger and thirst and have often gone without food; I have been cold and naked.
>
> —2 CORINTHIANS 11:23–27

The apostle Paul experienced a tremendous amount of physical persecution from religious leaders and government officials. His punishment was always unwarranted and, in some cases, was outright illegal.

And his suffering was not limited to physical pain—he also anguished emotionally. In the same chapter, Paul wrote, "Besides everything else, I face daily the pressure of my concern for all the churches" (v. 28). He founded several churches, but because of his missionary obligations, which required that he travel, he could not stay with the churches once they were established. Yet he felt responsible for their success whether he was present or absent. He rejoiced when the churches thrived, but grieved when they disregarded the precepts of the faith.

Paul experienced the emotional pain of separation when he said good-bye to the church leaders from Ephesus. (See Acts 20.) He told the elders of the church that he must leave them to go to Jerusalem; he confided that he knows going there will expose him to severe persecution, possibly death. He gave them advice on the manner in which they should lead the church, and then "he knelt down with all of them and prayed. They all wept as they embraced him and kissed him. What grieved them most was his statement that they would never see his face again. Then they accompanied him to the ship" (vv. 36–38).

Paul also knew the pain of rejection and betrayal. In his second letter to Timothy, he wrote:

> Do your best to come to me quickly, for Demas, because he loved this world, has deserted me and has gone to Thessalonica. Crescens has gone to Galatia, and Titus to Dalmatia...Alexander the metalworker did me a great deal of harm...At my first defense, no one came to my support, but everyone deserted me.
> —2 TIMOTHY 4:9–16

Paul wrote this letter to Timothy from death row, where he was awaiting execution. His friends abandoned him at the worst of times—they turned their backs while he sat, wrongly accused, in a cold, dark prison cell. Paul's circumstances were certainly painful, but no matter how profound his sorrow, there is no evidence to suggest that

Paul ever became depressed, despite his many trials and tribulations. Instead, we hear him declare:

> For I am convinced that neither death nor life, neither angels nor demons, neither the present nor the future, nor any powers, neither height nor depth, nor anything else in all creation, will be able to separate us from the love of God that is in Christ Jesus our Lord.
>
> —ROMANS 8:38–39

Paul chose to experience joy in the unconditional *agape* love of God. None of the typical symptoms of depression—loss of interest in daily activities, excessive fatigue, feelings of worthlessness, inability to concentrate—are found in the record of Paul's life. And even though he frequently contemplated death, he was neither suicidal nor was his preoccupation irrational. For Paul, the threat of death was real. His thoughts about dying involved the reality that he would eventually be martyred for his faith.

How do we apply the example of Paul's life to our own? How do we allow joy to shield us from depression, breaking any link between depression and obesity? It's not enough to acknowledge that joy is within us—any believer can do that. But, as with all the fruit of the Spirit, we must go beyond acknowledgment. We must choose to learn the keys to spiritual growth, allowing the fruit of the Spirit to be manifest in our lives.

THE KEYS TO JOY

As we have mentioned, Jesus desired for His disciples to have His joy. This is clear from His statement: "I have told you this so that my joy may be in you and that your joy may be complete" (John 15:11). Our desire is that we experience "complete joy." To do this we need to grasp the significance of Jesus' words.

Key #1: Personal relationship

Jesus was sharing with His disciples the nature of the believer's relationship with God the Father and with Himself, God the Son. He used the analogy of a vine, a gardener and a branch to describe our relationship with them:

> I am the true vine, and my Father is the gardener...
> I am the vine; you are the branches. If a man remains in me and I in him, he will bear much fruit; apart from me you can do nothing...As the Father has loved me, so have I loved you. Now remain in my love. If you obey my commands, you will remain in my love, just as I have obeyed my Father's commands and remain in his love. I have told you this so that my joy may be in you and that your joy may be complete.
> —JOHN 15:1, 5, 9–11

This passage reveals to us the first key to knowing the fruit of the Spirit of joy: that we believe in Christ. Jesus spoke these words the night before His death, giving the promise of His joy to His disciples. He was speaking to all of His disciples except for Judas, the betrayer, who had left the group earlier that evening to arrange for Jesus' arrest. So the disciples who remained were believers; they had faith in Christ, even though they were destined to turn their backs on Him—out of fear—after His arrest.

In order to receive the promise of "complete joy," we must enter into a faith-based relationship with Jesus, accepting Him as our Savior. Without this relationship—without first becoming branches of the vine—we can never know what it means to experience His "complete joy."

Key #2: Exalting God

The second key to experiencing complete joy is found in Psalm 100. This psalm opens with the appeal to "shout for joy to the Lord, all the earth." This is joy made manifest, an exuberance that is outwardly expressed. For some, it may seem difficult to give themselves to such candid expression.

But what is powerful enough to free us from our inhibitions? What can release us from the self-imposed need to maintain our composure and our false sense of dignity? What can excite us so much that we follow the scriptural command to "shout for joy"?

The answer is found in verse 3 of this psalm: "Know that the LORD is God. It is he who made us, and we are his; we are his people, the sheep of his pasture." The second key to joy lies in appreciating who God is. As we realize who God is, our response will be to exalt Him in praise and worship. The depth and magnitude of our joy depend on how fully we understand the wonder of who God is and His love toward us.

As Christians, we are not mere creations of God. Our status in His sight is not equivalent to the status of a rock or a tree; He has placed us on a higher level. The great and mighty God, the Creator of the universe, desires an intimate and personal relationship with every person He created. We are not insignificant to Him; He wants us to be identified with Him as "his people, the sheep of his pasture."

Tradition holds that when Cyrus the Great was born, his maternal grandfather dreamed that the child would one day rise up and take the Persian throne from him. The grandfather, overcome with fear and envy, ordered that the infant be put to death. But the servant who was assigned to kill the baby gave him to a shepherd instead.

So Cyrus the Great grew up believing that he was a shepherd's son and lived as a shepherd boy. Once he learned who he really was, his life changed dramatically. He began to live in a manner that reflected his true identity—that of a king. Eventually, King Cyrus *did* take the Persian throne. But this was only possible after he learned and appreciated who he really was.

Like King Cyrus, our lives are transformed when we begin to understand our true identity in Christ. And while we will never fully comprehend the richness of this relationship, as we *grow* in our understanding that wonderful destiny, our response will be one of pure, "shout about it" joy.

Key #3: Hope in God

We mentioned that the psalmist cried out, "Why are you downcast, O my soul? Why so disturbed within me?" (Ps. 42:5). His response to that question gives us another key to experiencing joy: "Put your hope in God, for I will yet praise him, my Savior and my God" (v. 5). He understood that hope changes discouragement to joy.

Hope is able to lift us out of despair and out of depression. It gives us vision beyond our circumstances, and it enables us to strive for the light at the end of the deepest and darkest tunnel. Hope, for the believer, is based on the knowledge that God is in control of all things—He's in control of our trials and tribulations, He's in control of our weight, and He's in control of our health.

Unfortunately, the term *hope* has been watered down, much like the term *love*. We use *hope* to describe some vague uncertainty that we are usually powerless to change: An expectant couple might hope for a boy; those planning a picnic will hope for pleasant weather; and an investor quite naturally hopes that stock prices work in his favor.

But the hope that gives us joy is not based on variables that are subject to change. To the contrary, the Christians' hope is grounded in our complete assurance and our unwavering certainty of God's promises—those which have been fulfilled and those that are yet unfulfilled.

His fulfilled promises are based in our knowledge that Jesus Christ is the Messiah, that He was murdered by crucifixion but rose from the dead, and that following His ascension into heaven, the Holy Spirit came to dwell in those who trust in Him.

Hope changes discouragement to joy.

Our hope that is yet unfulfilled rests in our knowledge that we as believers will spend eternity with our Lord.

The apostle Peter described this hope in an affirmation of joyful praise: "Praise be to the God and Father of our Lord Jesus Christ! In his great mercy he has given us new birth into a living hope through the resurrection of Jesus Christ from the dead, and into an inheritance that can never perish, spoil or fade—kept in heaven for you, who through faith are shielded by God's power until the coming of the salvation that is ready to be revealed in the last time" (1 Pet. 1:3–5).

When we experience adversity on earth, hope reminds us that trouble is nothing more than a temporal challenge. It pales in importance as we anticipate an eternity spent with God. And He has provided His love and joy in every challenge of life we face. As we focus on this spiritual reality, hope will begin to fill our hearts and minds and release the joy of the Lord to work in our lives.

Three

The Fruit of
the Spirit Is
Peace . . .

Better a dry crust with peace and quiet
than a house full of feasting, with strife.
—PROVERBS 17:1

My parents have told me stories about the Great Depression of the 1930s when poverty came quickly and hit hard. On October 29, 1929, without much warning, families that had plenty were faced with poverty so severe that going hungry was not uncommon. The lesson I've learned from hearing their account is that we cannot underestimate the value of intangible blessings.

One of those blessings is peace. Peace was a priceless commodity during the Great Depression. For those who experienced peace, the reality of financial ruin and the pain of poverty were much easier to bear. At a time when economic devastation destroyed relationships, produced fear and anxiety, and even provoked some to suicide, peace was (and still is) more precious than gold.

The Hebrew word for peace is *shalom*. It denotes a state of soundness, completeness and well-being. *Shalom* is used as a greeting in the Hebrew language, reflecting the desire that peace might abound in the life and relationships of the one being greeted. A sense of well-being is a powerful intangible blessing, one that many people, unfortunately, never experience.

Proverbs 17:1 gives an excellent word picture for the value of peace: "Better a dry crust with peace and quiet than a house full of feasting, with strife." The feasting referred to was the meal that was a result of a peace offering, also known as a fellowship offering. These involved animal sacrifices performed as an expression of gratitude to God for His fellowship.

Unlike other offerings, the peace offering required only the inner organs and fat of the animal to be burned. The family presenting the offering took the remainder of the animal home to eat. That meal symbolized their peaceful fellowship with God and right relationships with man. According to the Law of Moses, the whole animal was to be eaten on the same day that the offering was made. So it was a common practice for the family to host a great feast following the peace offering.

Some families were adhering to tradition by rote, participating in the ritual but missing its meaning. After going through the motions of the peace offering, they returned to homes that were anything but peaceful and engaged in a "fellowship" meal where no fellowship existed.

The peace offering was voluntary, and poor families who lacked the resources to host a large feast did not perform the sacrifice as often as rich families. From this understanding we grasp the significance of the proverb: If all the poor family had was a "dry crust" with peace, it was more valuable than a great feast held in a house full of strife.

There are situations in life that test the peace of the strongest and most mature of Christians. As we look at four of these difficult situations, we will discover how they can destroy our *shalom*—our soundness, completeness and sense of well-being. And we will discover how our lack of peace can influence the way we eat.

PEACE OR STRESS IN LIFE'S TRIALS

In the last chapter, we discussed the role that depression plays in obesity, how it can lead to overeating and how it destroys the motivation to exercise. Stress, either physical or psychological, is one of the triggers of depression. However, even in the absence of depression, stress can influence eating behavior. And, like those who eat because of depression, stress eaters will not gain control of their eating until they learn how to handle stress.

We typically feel stress when we are subjected to circumstances that we are powerless to change or control. When situations are under our control, they will not generate as much stress as when they are beyond our control. For example, traveling in a car moving ninety miles per hour can be stressful if you're sitting in the passenger's seat. If, on the other hand, you are the one doing the driving, then traveling so fast shouldn't create much stress at all. The situation is the same, but the level of stress is entirely different because of the sense of being in control.

While a certain degree of stress is an unavoidable part of living, extreme stress has a detrimental effect on our physical and mental health. Excessive stress depletes our bodies of nutrients, alters our hormonal and chemical balance and disturbs our sleep cycle. This kind of stress places us at risk for a number of diseases, ranging from heart disease to psychiatric disorders.

The consequences of stress are not universal, but vary from person to person. Those who are able to cope with stress are better off than those who don't cope well. The hallmark of an effective coping strategy is being able to stay relaxed no matter what the circumstances.

There's an old saying: *Anyone who can remain calm in this situation does not fully understand the situation.* But some people are able to remain calm, no matter how serious the circumstances. They simply don't allow the challenges of life to overwhelm them. Other people appear to be calm, but their calmness is artificially generated. This is what I call *pseudopeace,* a term I coined to describe a false sense of peace, the perception of tranquility that is not beneficial, but detrimental.

Pseudopeace is externally generated; it is derived through using substances that seem to help us cope. Some of these substances are illegal, like marijuana and heroin. The vast majority, however, are legal: prescription drugs, alcohol, tobacco and—in the case of the stress eater—food.

Pseudopeace is temporary at best, harmful at worst. The substance of choice does not provide a long-lasting sense of peace, but needs to be used over and over again. Those who rely on substances come to the point where they depend on them, a dependence that is either physical (as in the case with alcohol and narcotics, where withdrawal from the substance causes serious bodily changes) or psychological, as in the case with food. Whether physical or psychological, the end result is addiction—the most serious consequence of pseudo-peace.

People who become "stress" eaters

While the person addicted to alcohol, tobacco and drugs is sometimes censored for their vice, the food addict usually goes unnoticed. Food doesn't alter our mood or influence our thoughts so that we cannot function normally, as do alcohol and some drugs. And eating is a socially acceptable activity. But the tendency to turn to food in response to stress can be just as addictive as the tendency to pour a drink or light up a cigarette.

What makes a person a stress eater? From a physiologic standpoint, stress should actually decrease, rather than increase the appetite. Stress stimulates our bodies to release hormones that trigger what is known as the "fight or flight" response. Our pulse quickens, our breathing rate increases, and blood is shifted from our digestive system and other internal organs to the muscles in our arms and legs.

The changes these hormones bring about prepare us to fight against, or run away from, whatever is causing the stress. In either event—whether the choice is to fight or to run—it's clearly no time to eat. And this is why many people will *lose* their appetites in times of stress.

However, this is not true of stress eaters. No matter what the physiology, when the heat is on, they eat. Most stress eaters share a common trait that may explain their reaction to stress: They tend to closely monitor the way they eat. It's common knowledge that the world is made up of two types of people: those who regulate their eating, and those who don't. The latter eat whatever they want, whenever they want and however much they want without a great deal of thought. But if you're reading this book, chances are that you are not in that category. You are probably among the people who set up restraints when it comes to food. They are known as *inhibited* eaters, and they are prone to eat in response to stress.

Inhibited eaters, whether or not they are overweight, pay close attention to every aspect of eating. They count calories, measure portion sizes and make a conscious effort to control themselves for fear of overeating. But what happens when inhibited eaters are confronted with stress? It weakens their resolve. Stress will deplete them of the energy they need to monitor their eating. And once the restraints are removed, they overeat.

Not all forms of stress will unleash the inhibited eater. Most commonly it is the type of stress that violates his or her sense of self-worth. The stress generated by an escalating crime rate, the high cost of living or a broken-down car does not predispose the inhibited eater to overeat. These types of stressors don't challenge a person's sense of personal value.

On the other hand, the stress generated by the disparaging comments of a critical boss, the infidelity of a spouse or the disrespectful behavior of children *will* trigger overeating. Stress that comes from detraction and condemnation strikes the identity and diminishes the self-esteem. It acts as a painful trigger to out of control eating.

Stress eaters will often deny their problem or under-estimate the amount of food they actually eat. This denial may not be intentional—eating in response to stress is like a reflex; it's done without thinking.

When I encounter patients who deny that they eat under stress, but I suspect that they do, I will have them maintain a food journal for a few weeks. This requires them to keep a log of everything they eat, no matter how insignificant. They record the date, time and, most importantly, the circumstances associated with the eating. A typical page might have the following entries:

- Wed., 12 noon. Caesar salad, garlic bread, lemonade. Lunch.

- Wed., 2:00 P.M. Bag of potato chips, M & Ms. Failed final exam.

- Wed., 4:00 P.M. Coke and popcorn. Told Mom about failed exam.

If the journal is maintained honestly and consis-tently, it is always revealing. When we review it, we see right away those situations that prompted eating, and we usually find a strong connection between stress and impulse eating. It also provides a good estimate of the number of calories consumed each day—a piece of information that is valuable for those patients who swear they don't eat much.

Stress eaters use food to help them cope with the ups and downs of life. But food cannot provide true peace, only pseudopeace. True peace comes through a close relationship with God, whose Spirit gives us peace from within. The fruit of the Spirit of peace is an internal, not external, source of peace. It alone is able to keep us calm through any situation.

When we draw closer to God, He fills us with His peace. Scripture declares, "You will keep in perfect peace him whose mind is steadfast, because he trusts in you" (Isa. 26:3). As we become filled with God's peace, we will find that we don't need to resort to food or, for that matter, any substance to "help" our stress levels.

How Bible heroes beat stress

There is a dramatic example in the Old Testament of four young men who knew how to beat stress, though they probably did not use the term. Heroes of our childhood Bible stories, they suffered the kind of stress that violates personal identity, which could have caused them the same kinds of problems such stress causes today.

The Book of Daniel opens around 605 B.C., when Nebuchadnezzar became king of Babylon and soon thereafter besieged the city of Jerusalem. Along with the treasures he plundered from the temple in Jerusalem, Nebuchadnezzar also took with him some of the more intelligent and handsome young men to serve in his palace in Babylon.

Four of these young men were Daniel, Hananiah, Mishael and Azariah. Their Hebrew names had special meanings that reflected their trust in Jehovah God: Daniel, "God is my Judge"; Hananiah, "the Lord shows grace"; Mishael, "who is like God?" and Azariah, "the Lord helps."

Upon their arrival in Babylon, these young men were indoctrinated into the Babylonian lifestyle. They learned the customs and traditions and were even given

Babylonian names in an attempt to insure their full assimilation into this new culture. The Babylonian names assigned to them—Belteshazzar, Shadrach, Meshach and Abednego—honored the pagan gods of Marduk, Aku and Nebo.

So, along with being taken by force into a foreign land, they were pressured to take part in practices that were offensive to them and dishonoring to their God. Much of the lifestyle they were expected to assume was in direct violation to their principles and would require that they forsake their beliefs, their customs, their traditions—even their names. From the moment of their arrival, these young men experienced stressful circumstances, the kind of stress that strikes at the identity.

One thing expected of them was that they eat Babylonian food, even though some of these foods were forbidden by Jewish law. Daniel decided to negotiate with the ruler in charge for a diet that was more in keeping with Jewish tradition. He was successful, and the young men fared better on their diet than others did on the king's diet. But an occasion presented itself in which the other three—Shadrach, Meshach and Abednego—found themselves faced with a situation that was nonnegotiable.

King Nebuchadnezzar issued an edict that required everyone to honor a golden idol he built. The idol was enormous—ninety feet high and nine feet wide. At the sounding of a signal, people of all nations and languages were to fall down before the idol and worship it. For the Jews, this edict was a direct violation of the second commandment: "You shall not make for yourself an idol in the form of anything in heaven above or on earth beneath or in the waters below. You shall not bow down to them or worship them" (Exod. 20:4–5).

The penalty for failing to comply with the king's order was severe: Anyone who refused to worship the image would be thrown into a furnace and burned to death. But the three Hebrews chose to obey the God of Israel, no matter what the consequences. It wasn't long before their refusal was brought to the king's attention: "There are some Jews whom you have set over the affairs of the province of Babylon—Shadrach, Meshach and Abednego—who pay no attention to you, O king. They neither serve your gods nor worship the image of gold you have set up" (Dan. 3:12).

These young men found themselves facing the fiery furnace, an intense source of stress, as a result of their loyalty to their God and their Jewish identity. They were able to cope with this stress because of their relationship with God—a relationship that was established long before their confrontation with the furnace, one that was continually nurtured over the years. To avoid the stress on Nebuchadnezzar's terms would have required them to compromise their relationship with God. Their response to him shows us that compromise was not an option:

> O Nebuchadnezzar, we do not need to defend ourselves before you in this matter. If we are thrown into the blazing furnace, the God we serve is able to save us from it, and he will rescue us from your hand, O king. But even if he does not, we want you to know, O king, that we will not serve your gods or worship the image of gold you have set up.
> —DANIEL 3:16–18

They knew that no matter what the outcome—deliverance from the furnace or death by fire—they were the children of an omnipotent God who loved them. This confidence gave them a peace that made it possible for them to remain steadfast and unshaken, even when faced with death.

As you may know, their familiar story has a happy ending. And what was the outcome? It was divine protection and miraculous deliverance. God did not spare them from *experiencing* the stress—they did have to walk into that furnace. But He protected them from the adverse effects of the stress and eventually delivered them, completely unharmed, from the situation. King Nebuchadnezzar was even able to see the presence of God with them inside the furnace.

God was with them, and His presence allowed for them to come out of the situation unharmed. There weren't even any signs that they had been exposed to the stress: "The fire had not harmed their bodies, nor was a hair on their heads singed; their robes were not scorched, and there was no smell of fire on them" (Dan. 3:27). They entered the furnace in peace and exited it unscathed. This is the essence of the peace of God—it allows for us to face stress with confidence because we know that no matter what the outcome, God is in control.

Their reaction to the fiery trial revealed their level of trust in the Lord. Shadrach, Meshach and Abednego did not tremble in fear at the prospect of being thrown into the furnace, but they responded in a way that reflected their unwavering peace. And peace is what gave them the ability to cope effectively and appropriately with extreme stress. Even when offered a second chance, they courageously refused to bow down and worship the idol.

Shadrach, Meshach and Abednego exemplify the peace that the apostle Paul referred to in his letter to the Philippians: "Do not be anxious about anything, but in everything, by prayer and petition, with thanksgiving, present your requests to God. And the peace of God, which transcends all understanding, will guard your hearts and your minds in Christ Jesus" (Phil. 4:6–7).

> *We will never know the peace of God if we seek His face only in times of desperation.*

For these Hebrew boys, the peace of God did just that—it transcended understanding. They didn't weep, curse or wring their hands. They didn't show any signs of anger or defiance. The guards who were assigned to throw them into the furnace were overwhelmed by the heat and died. But even after the guards fell dead, Shadrach, Meshach and Abednego proceeded into the furnace on their own, never making any attempt to escape. They had an indescribable, incomprehensible peace that only comes through relationship with God.

When we look for peace in anything other than God, we cannot expect to exit the fiery furnaces of life untouched as the Hebrew boys did; rather, we will bear the scars from trusting in our source of pseudo-peace. God's peace builds us up; pseudopeace tears us down. Cigarettes, alcohol, drugs and even food may give momentary relief from stress, but they bring ultimate destruction to the body and the mind. The long-term effects of stress eating are directly linked to many illnesses involving diet and body weight. Turning to these and other sources of pseudopeace in times of stress will "burn us" far worse than anything we might suffer in the fiery furnaces of life.

You may ask, "What enables us to break our dependence on the things that bring pseudopeace?" The simple and effective answer is this: *knowing God.* Shadrach, Meshach and Abednego had a solid relationship with God that demonstrated their devotion to seeking Him. Their hearts were committed to following His precepts and pleasing Him. They sought the Lord with as much diligence when things were going well as they did when things were not.

We will never know the peace of God if we seek His face only in times of desperation. While He is certainly able to deliver us in our darkest hour, our desire to know Him ought to be equally fervent when there are no furnaces threatening us. Then when the threat comes, we can face it with the peace of God that has been nurtured in that relationship.

Only a deeply rooted relationship with God will give us the peace we need to handle the stress of life. The deeper our roots, the greater our peace. But deep roots don't develop from a sporadic and inconsistent fellowship. They come only from a ceaseless desire to know God and through personal prayer, meditation and Bible study. When we have the true peace of God, then the severity of the stress is irrelevant. Whether we are faced with a minor inconvenience or a true fiery furnace, we are able to cope with life's stressors when we rely on the presence and the peace of God.

PEACE OR PRESSURE IN PRIORITIES

There never seems to be enough time to accomplish everything we need to do. Consequently, we let ourselves get pulled in several different directions, and rather than experiencing peace, we feel pressure.

Americans are obsessed with time.

In the past few decades, time management has taken on a new level of significance. There are seminars conducted specifically for this purpose, attended by hundreds of people, all seeking to become better managers of time. The sponsors first lay the groundwork by pointing out the many ways we waste time. Then they go on to suggest that the best way to preserve our valuable time is through using their highly sophisticated daily planners, appointment books and hand-held gadgets. Major corporations pay for their executives to attend these seminars, expecting their investment to pay off with increased productivity and increased revenue—all because of optimally managed time.

Americans are obsessed with time. We have convinced ourselves that we will be better off if we can just speed up. By learning to do whatever it is we do just a little bit faster, we can squeeze a few more activities into an already frantic day.

True value priorities

When we feel that the twenty-four hours we've been allotted each day is simply not enough, we create a stressful atmosphere for ourselves. Unfortunately, the typical response to this stress is not to remove items from our "things to do" list—the most rational solution. Instead, we usually try to restructure our priorities in a way that we allow more time for those things we deem important and less time for everything else.

The things we perceive to be important are usually those things that give us an immediate sense of accomplishment. But some things that are vitally important do not give us that immediate gratification. For example, living a healthy lifestyle provides long-term benefits, not immediate rewards. So when we feel constrained by time, eating a healthy diet and engaging in regular exercise may fall a notch or two down on our list of priorities. In reality, this priority is more valuable than others we may have placed ahead of it.

For the average person, switching from an unhealthy diet to a healthy one requires a tremendous amount of time and effort. Learning new cooking techniques, planning nutritionally complete meals and becoming adept at reading food labels all require time—time that must be factored into an already tight schedule. And when the demands are high and time is limited, the temptation to resort to the old, unhealthy way of eating is strong. This is when we're prone to eat fast food—a guarantee for failing at losing weight.

One of the most visible icons of our fast-paced society is the fast-food restaurant. When they were first developed, fast-food restaurants were similar to full-service restaurants in that they provided indoor seating. The patron had the choice of eating there or ordering the food "to go." A few years later, the drive-through window emerged, which gave us the option of getting the food without even turning off the engine of the car.

As the pace of society continues to increase, so have the blueprints for fast-food restaurants. Now there are restaurant establishments that don't even have seats. They are designed to accommodate those who eat on the go, providing nothing but drive-through and walk-up service. It's fairly common to see a person steer with one hand and eat a burger with the other. It's so common that most cars are now equipped with built-in cup holders. And while this kind of eating on the run may be quick and convenient, the food is generally high in fat, high in calories and nutritionally deplete.

The temptation to sacrifice health for the sake of time is often irresistible. When I ask my patients who are struggling to lose weight how often they eat out each week, I am amazed at the answers I receive. Those patients with busy schedules may eat fast food as many as five times per week. The reason for this is invariably a perceived lack of time—they have determined that they simply cannot spare the time necessary to prepare a healthy meal. Instead, they rely on fast food for breakfast, lunch or dinner.

The real problem is not a lack of time. Time is a constant—twenty-four hours each day, no more, no less. So when we feel pressured by time constraints, it's not that time has grown more scarce; it's that we are trying to fit too many activities into an unyielding and constant variable. We try desperately to squeeze twenty-five hours worth of activities into a twenty-four-hour day. And when we fail, as we are destined to do, we think the problem will be solved by fine-tuning our time-management skills.

But there is no time-management seminar in the world that can create a twenty-five-hour day. The question we should ask ourselves is not, "What is the best way to manage my time?" Rather, it is, "What is the best way to structure my priorities?"

Mary and Martha syndrome

When I consider these questions, I am reminded of the biblical account of Mary and Martha, the two sisters of Lazarus, who were good friends of Jesus. (See Luke 10.) Mary and Martha were both confronted with a potentially stressful situation: Jesus stopped by for a visit. And even though Jesus was a friend of their family, He was nevertheless a very special guest—a VIP, so to speak. These sisters handled His visit in two completely different ways.

Martha directed her attention to the many things she felt she needed to accomplish, those things she perceived were important. I imagine that when she learned that Jesus was coming over, she immediately thought about all the things she'd need to do to make His visit as comfortable as possible.

We can't criticize Martha—at that time and in that culture good hospitality was important. But she ordered her priorities in a way that caused her undue tension and stress. She felt pressured to complete her many tasks: clean the house, prepare a meal and put everything in order. The Bible says that Martha was "distracted by all the preparations that had to be made" (Luke 10:40).

If Martha had an extra day or two to prepare for the visit, things might have been easier. But once it became clear that she didn't have enough time to prepare her home and listen to Jesus, she misplaced her priorities, opting to do the preparations instead of listening to the Master.

Eliminating some of the items from her "things to do" list would have been a better approach. Instead, Martha focused her attention on the tasks that gave short-term satisfaction—cleaning the house and preparing a meal. This decision, however, took time away from the one activity that would bring long-term results—listening to Jesus.

Mary handled the situation in an entirely different way. She knew the importance of showing good hospitality, but she decided that an opportunity to sit at the Lord's feet took precedence over a clean house. While the opportunity was the same for each sister, it was Mary who structured her priorities appropriately. She didn't just shift things around on her "things to do" list—she tore up the list.

Jesus' response to Martha's complaint that Mary was not helping her with her busyness makes it clear which sister was the better time manager:

> "Martha, Martha," the Lord answered, "you are worried and upset about many things, but only one thing is needed. Mary has chosen what is better, and it will not be taken away from her."
> —LUKE 10:41–42

Long-term priorities

It is important that we recognize our tendency to

respond like Martha to life's demands, and then discipline ourselves to behave more like Mary. We need to make sure that long-term priorities have the right place in our lives. This is especially true for women, who have a greater presence in the workplace now, compared to a generation ago, but are still charged with maintaining the home and raising children. Even with the most supportive, involved husband and the highest quality childcare, the challenge to meet the needs of both the workplace and the family is unrelenting. For the single parent, it can be overwhelming.

No matter how great the demands of life, it is crucial that we allow adequate time for the important things that don't seem to bring immediate satisfaction. Every Christian would agree that time should be set aside each day for prayer, meditation and Bible study. But since these activities may not generate as strong a sense of urgency as some of our other obligations, they are often neglected. We find ourselves rushing through a short psalm or speed-reading a page from a book of daily devotions, then concluding our "quality time with the Lord" with a quick, cursory prayer.

In that same way, the time we devote to our health also involves long-term results and, as such, tends to receive a priority rank much lower than those things that give us immediate results. For those people who are obese or overweight, or who have a medical condition that requires a lifestyle modification, this is a serious mistake. In the case of type 2 diabetes, for instance, it has been proven that keeping the blood sugar level tightly controlled will result in fewer long-term complications, such as kidney failure and blindness. This long-term goal of keeping the blood sugar controlled, however, requires daily attention and a significant allotment of time.

Even people who don't have illnesses and may presently have a normal body weight will benefit by devoting sufficient time toward maintaining their good health. A healthy diet and moderate exercise, for example, will yield the long-term results of protecting them from life-threatening diseases.

You may wonder what to do with all of your other obligations once you make the decision to commit adequate time to those things that provide long-term results. It may have occurred to you that if Martha stopped her cleaning and listened to Jesus, the following day she would be confronted with two days' worth of demands. The answer to this dilemma lies in eliminating some of our responsibilities.

I once heard a great piece of advice from Kay Coles James, a wise Christian woman and Senior Fellow of the Heritage Foundation: "Working women can do it all, we just can't do it all simultaneously." If we want to experience peace in our priorities, we must learn to guard our time and prune our list of responsibilities. One of the keys to doing this involves the issue of contentment.

PEACE AND CONTENTMENT

We have examined the potential power that stress has for robbing us of peace, which can result in overeating.

Then we looked at the problem of misplaced priorities that can contribute to an unhealthy lifestyle. Now we need to consider a root cause of both of these potential health hazards: *discontent.* Discontent is both the root cause for much of the stress we feel and the driving force that determines many of our priorities.

We learned that the Hebrew word for peace, *shalom,* denotes a state of completeness and contentment. We cannot fully appreciate the fruit of the Spirit of peace without learning to be content. Learning the secret of contentment that accompanies the fruit of the Spirit of peace will help us defeat the enemies to our health of stress and wrong priorities.

The value of contentment is grossly underestimated. Contentment is often overlooked in religious circles and usually ignored in secular ones. The idea of living in a state of total contentment is, in our society, a foreign concept. The fundamentals of the American Dream are expressed in a desire for *more* and *bigger,* even when the fewer and smaller things we already have will do. Discontent with what we have is considered normal for everyone pursuing the American Dream.

It is "normal" for men and women to accumulate vast stores of material possessions and to work diligently toward achieving a social or economic status that far exceeds the threshold of contentment. We don't ask ourselves how much is really enough, and we definitely can't be satisfied with the status quo. Only in recent years has this epidemic of discontent been recognized as a problem. There is now a growing movement to cure "affluenza," a term coined to describe this insatiable desire for material things.

Our need to learn contentment is taught throughout the Bible. In one of His more familiar parables, Jesus tells the story of a misguided man—a rich fool—who became obsessed with his material possessions:

> Then he said to them, "Watch out! Be on your guard against all kinds of greed; a man's life does not consist in the abundance of his possessions."
>
> And he told them this parable: "The ground of a certain rich man produced a good crop. He thought to himself, 'What shall I do? I have no place to store my crops.'
>
> "Then he said, 'This is what I'll do. I will tear down my barns and build bigger ones, and there I will store all my grain and my goods. And I'll say to myself, "You have plenty of good things laid up for many years. Take life easy; eat, drink and be merry."'
>
> "But God said to him, 'You fool! This very night your life will be demanded from you. Then who will get what you have prepared for yourself?'
>
> "This is how it will be with anyone who stores up things for himself but is not rich toward God."
> —LUKE 12:15–21

Contentment will protect us from becoming obsessed with material possessions and guard against our falling into a trap similar to that of the rich fool. He forfeited his relationship with God to pursue material wealth. Discontent is the fuel that keeps us striving perpetually for more and bigger and better. This insatiable drive will inevitably rob us of peace.

The apostle Paul warned Timothy, "The love of money is a root of all kinds of evil" (1 Tim. 6:10). In this same chapter he taught this young man that "godliness with contentment is great gain" (v. 6). We need to tell ourselves that not only is it OK to be content, it is a virtue for which we should strive, as the apostle Paul also taught.

In his letter to the Philippians, Paul notes, "I have learned to be content whatever the circumstances. I know what it is to be in need, and I know what it is to have plenty. I have learned the secret of being content in any and every situation, whether well fed or hungry, whether living in plenty or in want. I can do everything through him who gives me strength" (Phil. 4:11–13). Paul did not define himself by his circumstances or his possessions. He was able to live a life of complete satisfaction because he focused not on what he *had* but on what the Lord empowered him to *do*. This was his *secret* of being content. He was completely detached from his material possessions, which allowed him the freedom to enjoy life's perks when he had them, but not *sweat it* when he didn't. The end result was a life that glorified God.

Contentment and body weight

How does contentment relate to body weight? In a few ways. First, most people are motivated to climb the corporate ladder primarily for two reasons: more money and recognition or status. The downside to these motivations is that career advancement is time consuming and invariably causes stress—two risk factors we've already discussed that can lead to overeating and poor nutrition. And in religious, political or even humanitarian circles, the drive to advance a cause can also create a stressful lifestyle. For those who have a weight problem, this syndrome of perpetual discontent spells disaster.

Second, contentment relates to body weight for those who are primarily concerned about their appearance, even if they don't have a weight problem at all. These are people, most commonly women, who torment themselves in an effort to lose weight simply because they are discontent with their appearance.

These people are always on a diet. Everything they eat is first evaluated for its calorie count and fat content, and they set unnecessary limits on what foods are permissible for them. Consequently, they rob themselves of the fun and spontaneity of eating and become virtual prisoners to their plates.

Unfortunately, this form of discontent begins at an early age. Young girls begin discussing diets as early as the third grade. Some of them actually begin to restrict their eating at this age, even when their body weight is normal. So, long before reaching adolescence, their desire is for their bodies to look like that of a fashion model or—worse yet—a Barbie doll. This spirit of discontent can lead to serious psychiatric disorders such as anorexia nervosa and bulimia nervosa. It can also cause physical problems. For example, if calcium-rich foods such as milk and cheese are eliminated during the growing years, then osteoporosis is sure to develop later in life.

Discontent also plagues the overweight person who is genuinely interested in losing weight. I was surprised to learn that many of my obese patients didn't like to exercise because they were afraid to be "caught exercising." They avoid the health club, the park and wherever else they could go to exercise because they are ashamed of their appearance. And they fear they might be ridiculed or laughed at if seen in a jogging suit, leotards or swimwear.

For my troubled friends, I want to encourage you to discard your sense of discontent. When the Bible says that we are created in the image and likeness of God, there are no qualifiers that relate to body weight. When the Spirit of God lives within us and we receive His peace, we can enjoy a sense of contentment regardless of our appearance or body weight.

The Lord gives His peace to a 300-pound person in the same way that He gives it to a person with a 150-pound frame. So the notion that says "I'll feel content *when* I reach my goal" should be replaced with "I can be content *while* I reach my goal."

Contentment, not complacency

Contentment is not synonymous with complacency. I regularly encounter men and women who resist my advice that they lose weight on the grounds that they are "content" with their appearance. And while I am happy about their healthy dose of self-esteem, I still recommend weight loss for anyone who is overweight or obese, even more strongly for those with weight-related medical conditions.

We cannot allow ourselves to be content with a body weight that will cause excess illness and premature death. This is not the contentment that comes through the fruit of the Spirit of peace. Instead, it indicates a state of ignorance, apathy or denial.

Resisting the truth of our need to live a healthy lifestyle and ignoring the parameters that indicate health are not a sign of contentment. Rather, they indicate a need to face ourselves honestly and to embrace a willingness to change. One reason we allow ourselves to get comfortable with the status quo, even when the status quo is making us sick, is that we have an underlying fear of change.

PEACE IN INEVITABLE CHANGE

One of the most difficult things about losing weight is accepting the inevitability of the need to change. There is comfort in the familiar. This is the reason why change is not easy—just thinking about breaking old habits, even bad habits, can generate anxiety.

For example, the workplace is full of people who are discontent with their jobs. But they remain in those jobs for years, sometimes even decades, never venturing out to learn a new trade or master a skill that would enable them to enter a more enjoyable career. The prospect of change causes such a sense of insecurity that they choose to continue doing work they dislike rather than risk change.

Even when a change is implemented, the tendency to regress back to the old way of doing things never seems to go away. This is why New Year's resolutions are so often doomed to failure. Our initial enthusiasm for the positive change wanes with time, and the "bad habit" recurs before the end of January.

Phases of change

Several years ago, James Prochaska wrote an article in

which he described how people go about changing an undesirable behavior.[1] He observed that when we try to break a harmful or addictive habit, including overeating, we unconsciously proceed through five different phases. Each phase draws us closer to the point where we are totally successful in reaching our goal. You may identify the phase you are presently going through in your desire to reach your goal of permanent weight loss.

Pre-contemplative. The first phase of change is called the *pre-contemplative* stage. People in this stage have not yet acknowledged that they even have a problem. If they go through the motions of changing the behavior, it's usually to appease someone else—not because they are genuinely interested in changing. For example, an employer might threaten to fire an alcoholic employee unless he starts attending Alcoholics Anonymous meetings. The employee will go through the motions and attend AA, not because he acknowledges a drinking problem, but because he fears unemployment.

Many overweight and obese people stay in this first stage out of ignorance—they are simply unaware that their excess weight imposes a risk to their health. But if you are reading this book, I'll assume that you've proceeded beyond the pre-contemplative stage and are, at the minimum, in the second phase of change (unless, of course, someone who loves you and desires that you improve your health has coerced you into reading it).

Contemplative. The second phase of change is the *contemplative* stage. In this stage there is acknowledgment of a need for change, but no steps are taken to make it happen. This phase can last for years; some have spent their lifetimes contemplating a lifestyle change. A good example is the pack-a-day cigarette smoker who reads the Surgeon General's warning, agrees with it, admits to himself that he should quit and then proceeds to light up.

Preparation. The third phase is known as the *preparation* phase. The light has dawned; a decision is made. And the person begins to consider how to make the necessary change. Plans for action are considered and choices made to implement the necessary changes.

Action. Preparation is closely followed by the *action* phase. People in these two phases have taken steps, however small, toward changing their behavior. If you are reading this book because you sincerely want to lose weight or because you want to know how your spiritual life influences your physical condition, you probably belong in one of these two phases—you're either preparing for change, or you are actively working at it.

Maintenance. The final stage of the cycle of change is *maintenance*. Once the change is implemented, our improved health requires that we maintain our new lifestyle for the long term. In my opinion, this is the most challenging of all five phases. The challenge is twofold; it involves an *internal* test and an *external* test.

In the case of weight loss, the inner test comes from having to resist the temptation of returning to wrong eating habits and the need to stay motivated enough to engage in regular exercise. The external test comes in dealing with the negative expectations of others. All eyes seem to be on the person in the maintenance phase. Many of those eyes are expectantly waiting for the weight to return.

The goal: termination. It's not uncommon—in fact, it's expected—for people to cycle through these phases of change over and over again. For example, the average cigarette smoker has tried to quit more than once. With each successful attempt, he proceeds through the five stages of change, but falls back to one of the initial phases when he resumes the habit. Ideally, he'll eventually reach the point where he is completely delivered from smoking. When that happens he has reached the successful goal of termination. This sometimes, but not always, requires a person to cycle through the five phases several times. We will discuss this ultimate freedom more in the next chapter.

Changes necessary for weight loss

No matter how difficult it is to accept, the truth is that in order to lose weight and keep it off, something must change. And the change must be permanent. Typically, it is not *one* change that is necessary for successful weight loss, but *three*:

- Our attitude toward food

- The types and amounts of food we eat

- Our commitment to physical activity

Assuming that, because you are reading this book you have passed the pre-contemplation stage that denies any need of change, it will be helpful to highlight some things you may encounter during the next phases of change to reach your contemplated goal for weight loss.

Hopefully you are contemplating change before you

have been diagnosed with any of the diseases for which you are predisposed as a result of overweight or obesity. Some weight-related medical conditions take years to reach the point where they are detectable by screening tests or where they produce obvious symptoms. The onset of these diseases can be delayed, or in some cases entirely prevented, if lifestyle changes that include weight loss are implemented early on—long before a diagnosis is made.

Some typical responses for the contemplator who is acknowledging his or her need of change are anger and frustration. It takes courage to admit to a problem for which there seems no clear or easy solution. During this contemplative phase it is easy to fall back on lame excuses that threaten to take the contemplator back to the pre-contemplative state of denial.

Overweight people in this second phase of change can become paralyzed from a lack of self-confidence. They don't deny that obesity is a problem, but their uncertainty in their ability to succeed in their weight loss goals prevents them from even trying. This is especially common in people who have weight cycled—repeating the five phases of change—and find themselves back in phase two after repeated attempts to lose weight. Their fear of experiencing yet another failure will keep them from venturing beyond this phase of contemplation one more time.

Allowing the peace of God that passes understanding (Phil. 4:7) to be released within us will give us courage to move on to the third phase of change—preparation. That happens as we follow the scriptural instruction, "Do not be anxious about anything, but in everything, by prayer and petition, with thanksgiving, present your requests to God" (v. 6). Asking for and receiving the help of God will turn our impossibilities into realities. His desire for us is health, peace and contentment, and He will help us achieve those goals.

For weight loss, the preparation phase is usually very practical. It's when we accomplish those things that get us ready to lose weight—learning to interpret food labels, getting comfortable with new cooking techniques, joining a health club and fitting exercise into our daily schedule. Most importantly, we prepare ourselves spiritually, acknowledging that the Lord we serve is more powerful than any force that might tempt us to neglect our health.

The action phase closely follows the preparation phase, as we have mentioned. The action phase of losing weight is an uplifting time. As we approach our weight loss goals, there is a satisfying sense of being in total control. This, along with the accompanying physical benefits of weight loss—increased level of energy, fewer aches and pains and improved sleep—makes the action phase the most exhilarating.

Often the exhilaration is short lived, however, because what follows is the fifth and most challenging phase of change—maintenance. Statistics show that long-term success of weight loss is very low because of the rate of failure in this maintenance phase of change. Only 5 to 10 percent of all people who successfully lose weight are able to keep it off for longer than five years. Most go on to become "yo-yo dieters" who lose weight and regain it over and over again.

Why is the maintenance of yearned-for weight loss

goals so challenging? Much of the failure is due to an inability to adapt to the new lifestyle required for maintaining a healthy weight. We simply cannot stop yearning for the harmful eating habits of the past.

For example, when we feel compelled to eat unhealthy portions simply because food is abundant in a social setting or at a party, we are setting ourselves up to fail in the maintenance phase. One way to gauge whether your eating is in response to hunger or just food availability is to observe how you behave at "all you can eat" restaurants. If you can go into one of these facilities and stop eating at the point you feel full, then you are well prepared for the maintenance phase. If, on the other hand, you have the tendency to go back to the buffet line again and again just because it is there, you may expect to have trouble keeping the weight off that you have lost.

Typically what sets us up for failure in the mainte-nance phase is that foods that were once eaten with abandon are the same ones we crave once the "diet" is over. The term *diet* has fallen out of favor for good reason—too many consider it a time of temporary deprivation, which, if endured until the end, reim-burses us with a ticket to indulge in all our old eating habits.

Success in the maintenance phase, however, requires that we abandon this concept of temporary deprivation and accept dietary changes that are permanent. It doesn't mean that high-fat, high-calorie foods can never be eaten again. But they will only be enjoyed in moderation—infrequently and in small amounts.

It will help us to make a conscious effort to associate

these harmful foods with oppression that results in obesity and let them become symbols of bondage to poor health. Then it won't be as difficult to limit them from our diets. They should serve as constant reminders of the many undesirable and potentially life-threatening consequences of being overweight.

Rather than focusing on the foods we *can't* eat, we must focus our attention on the wonderful foods we *can* eat to nourish our bodies, as well as on the benefits of losing weight. A lower blood pressure, a lower cholesterol level and better control of type 2 diabetes will increase the chances of living a longer, healthier life. By relying on the power of the Holy Spirit to keep us in perfect peace, we will enjoy victory in the maintenance phase and will be delivered from our cruel bondage to food.

Four

The Fruit of
the Spirit Is
Patience . . .

The end of a matter is better than its beginning, and patience is better than pride.

—ECCLESIASTES 7:8

After our fourth child was born, my husband and I decided that we needed to move into a larger home. It was a practical decision, not fueled by discontent or affluenza. Neither of us is a show-off, and we have no desire to "keep up with the Joneses"—we just needed more space. So when the baby was almost a year old, we moved into a bigger house. The new house wasn't just larger on the inside; it also had a large backyard. This extra backyard space gave me a burning desire to start a garden.

I had very little experience with gardening. As a little girl, I'd help my mother plant flowers each spring, and for a few years we even planted vegetables. But the kind of flower and vegetable beds I envisioned would require a level of skill and expertise that far exceeded my childhood experience. So I began reading books and watching television programs devoted to gardening, and I soon discovered that there was much more to it than simply buying a flat of marigolds, digging a hole in the ground to put them in and hoping for rain.

In my studies I learned about annuals, perennials and bulbs. I learned about hardiness, zones and blooming times. I learned about fertilizers, weed-killers, insecticides and mulch. I learned about the various soil types—clay soil, sandy soil and the coveted loam soil. I learned how to till the soil and how to amend the soil with organic matter like compost and peat moss.

When I felt that I was finally ready to plant, I looked at a catalog and found a picture of the flowerbed of my dreams. The bed contained nine different plants that bloomed at different times of the season, so I could enjoy flowers from the beginning of spring until late fall. Along with a detailed description of each plant, the catalog also provided a diagram of the size and shape of the flowerbed and where each plant should be placed. I phoned in my order, and my husband and I took on the task of clearing out a fifteen- by five-foot plot of earth. This meant we had a huge amount of sod to remove and ground to till so that we would be ready for the arrival of my plants.

I didn't know what to expect, but having prepared such a large amount of soil, I was surprised when the box of plants arrived at how small it was. I was even more surprised at its sparse contents. Most of the plants were delicate leaves and fragile stems planted in two-inch plastic containers. But nearly half of the plants had no green at all—they were just clumps of brown, dry, gnarled roots inside of sealed plastic bags.

Feeling disappointment well up inside, I went back to the catalog and read the fine print. Sure enough, it clearly stated that I shouldn't expect to enjoy the garden that was pictured for at least three seasons. The flowerbed of my dreams was to begin with a few tiny roots, strategically placed in 60 square feet of earth. In spite of all the information I had gained from my studies, the first *real* lesson I learned in gardening was the lesson of *patience*.

After I realized that the flowerbed I selected would require a minimum of three years to materialize, I had to make a simple choice: to wait patiently or to wait impatiently. I could patiently nurture and cultivate those delicate plants, or I could throw up my hands at the dismal prospect of waiting, which would result in a waste of my investment of time, labor and money.

I did not have a choice to wait or not to wait. My choice was limited to my *reaction* to the inevitable wait required to have my beautiful garden. If I chose the right reaction—patience—"the end of the matter" would truly be better than the beginning. A lush and colorful flowerbed patiently cultivated would be much more aesthetically appealing than a bed of weeds the bed would produce if left on its own. The three years would ultimately pass regardless of my choice, but my choice determined the end result—a bed of flowers or a bed of weeds.

One of the most difficult things to accept when it comes to weight loss is the need to wait patiently. A typical scenario is the woman in her late thirties or early forties who comes to me for assistance in losing weight. This typical patient might tell me that she did not have a weight problem as a child or even during her adolescent years, but that she has steadily gained weight as an adult. Together we estimate that she's gained about five pounds per year and is about fifty to sixty pounds heavier than she was on her wedding day.

And then comes her request. She wants to lose forty pounds in six weeks before leaving for the Caribbean or attending her class reunion. She wants my opinion about some fad diet or liquid diet she's read about, or she wants to know what I think about using "colon cleansers" or taking pills designed to boost the metabolism. She seems oblivious to the fact that it took over a decade for her to accumulate the weight—she just wants it all gone in a month or two.

As we cultivate the fruit of the Spirit of patience in our lives, it will help us to hold fast to the "end of the matter." As Solomon says in this proverb from the Book of Ecclesiastes, "The end of a matter is better than its beginning." When we become impatient (as we are prone to do), we set ourselves up for failure and disappointment. Learning to yield to the Holy Spirit to empower us to be patient involves not only a willingness to wait, but also a willingness to endure whatever trials are destined to come our way while we wait.

PATIENCE FOR RECEIVING DELIVERANCE

In our discussion of the five phases required for successful change, we mentioned that often people repeat these cycles endlessly, never ultimately enjoying freedom from the bondage they are trying to break. We concluded that the last phase—maintenance—is without question the most difficult phase to master.

The thought of spending the rest of our lives in the maintenance phase is not very encouraging. But don't get discouraged, because there is hope for exiting this *cycle* of change altogether, as we have mentioned. While the maintenance phase is the last point in the cycle of change, it is possible (and desirable) to reach a point whereby you exit the cycle altogether. Your ultimate goal is to achieve *termination*. Termination is characterized by living in a freedom where you are no longer burdened with the tendency to fall back into the old lifestyle.

In the secular world, the term *recovered* describes those who reach the termination phase. But for the Christian, the termination phase is more accurately expressed by the term *deliverance*. The time element required between maintenance and termination, or deliverance, varies for different people. The Lord will keep you in the maintenance state until you learn what will prevent you from falling back into the old lifestyle.

King David's deliverance

In the fortieth psalm, King David wrote:

> I waited patiently for the LORD; he turned to me and heard my cry. He lifted me out of the slimy pit, out of the mud and mire; he set my feet on a rock and gave me a firm place to stand. He put a new song in my mouth, a hymn of praise to our God. Many will see and fear and put their trust in the LORD.
>
> —PSALM 40:1–3

David uses a very descriptive metaphor to equate whatever difficulty he was experiencing to being stuck in a pit of slimy mud. His problem was a hindrance; it was distressing, and it kept him in bondage. And while the passage does not specify the actual cause for his distress, it must have troubled him for a prolonged period of time for he was required to *wait patiently.* The good news is that God responded to David's cry to deliver him from his unpleasant condition after he waited patiently for the Lord.

Why did the Lord require David to wait before he was delivered from the pit? And why are we required to wait in difficult circumstances, stuck in our own pits of life? Perhaps God has a different answer to those questions for each of His children. But one common element in the purpose of waiting is that there is a valuable lesson that can only be learned through a pit experience.

In those difficult "pit" experiences we are inclined to focus our attention on God as the source of our help. It is there that we receive from God the guidance and discipline that we would otherwise miss. And because of His love for us, God will make us stay in the mud until we have received all the "benefits" of the mud—He will keep us there as long as it takes us to grow into His grace for our need.

The obsession pit

So what "pits" entrap overweight and obese people? What stumbling blocks are as tenacious as mud that grips like quicksand? What is it that has the potential of holding us prisoners to a phase of the cycle of change, when what we desperately want is to exit the cycle and enjoy true deliverance?

For many overweight and obese people, the answer lies in food obsession and food addiction. According to Webster's dictionary, an obsession is *the domination of one's thoughts or feelings by a persistent idea, image, desire or feeling.* In the case of food, we do not easily identify obsession as a problem, because eating is one of America's favorite pastimes. As a culture we have obsessed over food to such an extent that it seems normal to be preoccupied with eating.

I have a friend who once had a visitor from Ghana in her home. A few days into his stay, having had the opportunity to observe many aspects of American life, he politely but frankly asked her, "Why do Americans eat so much?" She was taken aback by the question, not having considered that we do. The answer to the question, however, is crystal clear: It is because we are obsessed with food.

Women are especially susceptible to food obsessions because we are bombarded in media and advertising with multiple, often conflicting, messages about food. A typical women's magazine may have any number of articles on proper nutrition, staying healthy and losing weight. But the cover of that same magazine might display a picture of a multi-layered chocolate cake, with the promise of the recipe for this "decadent dessert" inside. Leafing through the magazine invariably reveals page after page of messages related to food—advertisements, coupons, recipes and articles. The end result of these media blitzes is an excessive preoccupation with food that pervades our culture.

You may ask the astute question, *How is it possible to lose weight without thinking about food?* In spite of our cultural obsession with food, we must keep in mind that there is nothing innately wrong with thinking about food. In fact, you *must* put some thought into following a healthy, well-balanced diet. But there is a vast difference between normal thought processes and an obsession.

For the sake of illustration, consider people with insomnia. They typically spend an excessive amount of time thinking about sleep: what will induce sleep, what will hinder sleep and how to improve the quality and the quantity of sleep. Long before bedtime, they think about what time they should retire, whether it would be better to go to bed a little earlier or a little later. It doesn't matter where they are or what they're doing; they constantly think about some aspect of sleep.

Most likely, people with insomnia have friends or relatives who have never had trouble falling asleep. And these friends may have a difficult time relating to this constant preoccupation with sleep. For them, sleep is not something you think about—it just happens. They are convinced that if their suffering friend spent less time thinking about sleep—that is, if he or she stopped obsessing about it—they would have fewer problems.

In the same way that our hypothetical insomniac spends an excessive amount of time thinking about sleep, some overweight and obese people demonstrate an excessive preoccupation with every aspect of food— where to do the grocery shopping, what to prepare, what snacks to buy and what to do with leftovers.

People who obsess about food in their thoughts also tend to talk about food too much. I have a friend who has struggled to lose weight for many years. She has tried several diet plans with the same results—short-term success, long-term regain. Her weight problem won't be resolved until she addresses the root of her problem— her food obsession. How is it that I am sure she's obsessed with food? By listening to her conversation.

When my friend visits my home, right after we greet each other, her conversation usually involves a question like, "What are you cooking for dinner tonight?" When I tell her, she continues to question me about how I plan to prepare my entree, what side items I'll serve with it and what kind of dessert I plan to serve. Her conversation betrays the thoughts that are uppermost in her mind—food.

We must recognize the seriousness of our obsessions in order to allow God to rescue us from these "pits." Jesus taught us:

> Do not worry about your life, what you will eat or drink; or about your body, what you will wear. Is not life more important than food, and the body more important than clothes?... For the pagans run after all these things, and your heavenly Father knows that you need them. But seek first his kingdom and his righteousness, and all these things will be given to you as well.
> —MATTHEW 6:25, 32–33

As children of God, we should never be anxious about our basic needs because the Lord, our heavenly Father, has promised to provide them. Even though this passage is directed primarily to those who worry about whether or not there will be *enough* to eat, it can also be applied to people who have plenty to eat but obsess about it. Our preoccupation with these personal needs denies our Father's tender concern for us, and it takes our minds off of His will for us to seek His kingdom and His righteousness.

The apostle Paul understood our right priorities to seek the kingdom of God and to honor God in our bodies when he declared, "'Everything is permissible for me'—but I will not be mastered by anything. 'Food for the stomach and the stomach for food'—but God will destroy them both" (1 Cor. 6:12–13). He refused to be mastered by his physical appetites that were not eternal, instructing us to honor God in our body (v. 20).

Obsession is sin. Anything that absorbs our attention to this excessive degree has become too important in our lives; it is an idol that threatens to replace God. When we are obsessed with food, instead of eating to live our lives for the glory of God, we live to eat. How can we free ourselves from obsessive thinking and speaking that bring destruction into our lives and hinder our relationship with God?

Secrets for guarding against addiction

In Paul's second epistle to the Corinthians, he says to "take captive every thought to make it obedient to Christ" (2 Cor. 10:5). This verse gives us an important secret to guarding against obsession—we protect ourselves by choosing to keep our thoughts in agreement with the mind of Christ. It is important to realize that through the work of the Holy Spirit we have power to control the things we think about. As we choose to yield to His power, nothing will be able to preoccupy a Christian's mind to the point of obsession.

Overcoming a food obsession is important because obsession leads to addiction. *Addiction* is defined by Webster as "the state of being enslaved to a habit or practice or to something that is psychologically or physically habit-forming, to such an extent that its cessation causes severe trauma." What we think about, we act upon. When we won't stop thinking and talking about food, we are opening the door to food addiction—the state in which a person is enslaved by the act of eating.

The hallmark of an addiction is a loss of control, an inability to resist that thing that enslaves our appetites, even when we are fully aware of the adverse consequences involved in yielding. A food addiction is particularly difficult to treat. Unlike an addiction to tobacco, alcohol or drugs, a food addiction is prone to go unrecognized, as we mentioned, because eating is a legal, socially acceptable activity that is necessary to sustain life. Even family members and friends—those who would quickly notice a drug or alcohol problem—might fail to recognize our food addiction.

Obsession and addiction will keep us from experiencing total deliverance from the grip of food. They are enemies lurking between the maintenance stage in the cycle of change and termination—the door to freedom. To return to the analogy of our psalm, they are "slimy pits" that keep us in bondage. Deliverance from these pits requires more than just identifying the obsession and addiction as the root of the problem, though that is necessary.

Our deliverance cannot be expected to happen "instantaneously" or overnight. For us to enjoy complete freedom from obsessions and addictions, we will have to allow the Holy Spirit to cultivate the fruit of patience in our lives. Jesus declared, "In your patience possess ye your souls" (Luke 21:19, KJV). The New International Version says, "By standing firm you will gain life." Our souls involve our intellect, our will and our emotions. As we learn to yield our minds, wills and desires to the Holy Spirit, He will empower us to take every thought captive and make dramatic changes in our priorities and our lifestyle—it is a process that requires patience.

The secret of our deliverance rests in our willingness to submit to this divine process that will involve deep *repentance* for our sin and learned *dependence* on the power of the Holy Spirit.

The repentance factor. Repentance is crucial to our deliverance from obsession and addiction, though it is often overlooked or entirely avoided. Repentance basically means that we agree with God that our behavior is wrong. It is acknowledging our sin and agreeing that the sin is a problem that must be removed. As simple as this may sound, many Christians never receive deliverance because of their failure to repent for their sin. Some have the false notion that repentance is a one-time act that does not have to be repeated, even in the face of subsequent sinful behavior.

What would keep a person from repenting? Pride and self-righteousness. To repent requires humility; the humble person lives a lifestyle of repentance. Rather than humbly acknowledge our sin through confession, we have a tendency to justify the sin and vindicate ourselves in our own eyes.

In the problem of overweight and obesity, my experience is that most people are *not* humbly repentant; they staunchly defend their behavior. Even when that behavior involves the sin of gluttony, which is idolatry, patients are willing to defend their lifestyle. Their idolatry, which is the foundation of addiction, must be repented of if they hope to be delivered from their weight problem.

If your comments about your weight never reflect any degree of personal accountability ("I don't know why I can't seem to lose weight," or "I really don't eat that much"), then it's likely that a failure to repent is holding you back from deliverance.

I used to believe that total deliverance would be the immediate result of repentance. And that has been the experience of some. Surely God has the power to take us immediately from repentance, the point where we agree with Him that our behavior is sinful, to the point of complete deliverance where we never again desire to engage in the sin. However, though I am confident that God is able to instantly deliver us, my observation is that it usually doesn't happen that way. And, as is always the case, the problem is not with God, but with us.

Instead of instant deliverance, most people go through a period of "walking in repentance." There is agreement with God that the problem is a sin, but there is still the tendency to stumble and fall back into the sin. Full deliverance takes us beyond the point of being constantly prone to stumble. When we enter the termination phase, we are no longer walking in sinful behavior that requires our constant repentance (that is, repeating the cycle of stumbling and repenting) because we are free and victorious, fully delivered from the desire to commit the sin. The secret to complete deliverance that stands between walking in repentance and the termination state is acknowledging our dependence upon God.

The dependence factor. Too often, after taking the step of repentance, our first response is to try to overcome the problem in our own strength. We become self-confident, assuming that nothing is so serious that it can't be conquered through will power and sheer determination. The magnitude of the problem is minimized while the sense of self-sufficiency is maximized. The end result is that instead of achieving full deliverance, we enter the phase of walking in repentance while still struggling to be completely removed from the slimy pit.

But God has a lesson for us to learn while we struggle in that slime. And the lesson is simple: We can't do it on our own. Just when we think that the food addiction is under control, just when we think we have a handle on those obsessive thoughts about food, and just at the moment we feel we are stepping out of the pit, something will predictably happen that causes us to slip right back into the slime. And we find that after vowing to never again buy chocolate, we eat a whole box in one sitting, or after swearing to eat beef only in moderation, we indulge in an inch-thick 12-ounce steak. The lusts of the flesh will invariably prevail when we rely on our own strength.

God will not pull us out of the pit if we are convinced we can get out of our mess on our own. But when we cry out to Him with a pure heart, when we come to Him broken and contrite, acknowledging our weaknesses and admitting that in and of ourselves we are powerless, then He will show himself faithful, pull us out of the pit and set us on solid ground. Deliverance will not come without humble repentance and our acknowledgment of our total dependency on God. We must accept the reality that it is through the merciful forgiveness and the grace and power of God we are able to overcome.

OVERCOMING THE EVIDENCE OF THE PIT

It would be nice to say that the challenge ends with our deliverance. But it doesn't. While deliverance releases us from the grip of the pit and establishes us on the firm foundation of Christ, it does not remove the *evidence* of our time spent inside the pit. No one comes out of a pit smelling like roses. And even though we rejoice that our feet are planted on solid ground, we can't ignore the obvious: We're covered with mud and smell like slime. Specifically, our body is still over-weight because of our past behavior. Patience continues to be a fruit of the Spirit that must be matured and manifested in our lives in order to reach our ultimate goal—permanent weight loss.

If we look at the experience of an alcoholic or drug addict at the point of their deliverance, more often than not they find that their lives are in a state of total chaos. My husband has a very close friend who spent over twenty years in the pit of substance abuse. When he was in his mid-forties, he called upon the Lord and was born again. Then after his conversion, he spent another few years in the pit of addiction, trying over and over again to pull himself out by his own strength.

When he finally understood what it meant to be totally dependent upon Christ, the Lord released him from the bondage of addiction, and he has been drug free, alcohol free and tobacco free ever since. But his life was a mess. The evidence of the pit was overwhelming—broken relationships, missed opportunities and financial troubles. And facing his situation was especially painful because drugs and alcohol no longer clouded his perceptions.

The good news is that my husband's friend was able to get through this painful time by allowing patience to work in his life. He accepted the fact that the destruction in his life did not happen overnight and that the restoration process would involve some time as well.

Patience with the process

Deliverance from a food addiction is similar—the number when you step on the scale reads exactly the same at the point of your deliverance as it did when you were in the pit of obsession and addiction. Though you can rejoice that the spiritual bondage is gone, the pounds will remain, at least for a while. If there is no commitment to grow in patience, feelings of discouragement with the "evidence" may be overwhelming. Without patience, all of the exuberance that was part of the deliverance experience will give way to discouragement and despair.

Patience is required because weight loss is a slow process. As we get older, the body's rate of metabolism slows down, making it all the more difficult to lose those pounds that were so easy to gain during our younger years. It also requires patience to continue with an exercise program and adhere to a healthy diet when the results we want to see will not be evident for weeks, maybe even months. And it takes patience to guard against the ever-present temptation of the fad diet or "quick-fix" weight loss plan.

Patience with prejudice

It also takes patience to deal with the prejudices and stereotypes directed at overweight and obese people. Society still maintains a strongly negative attitude toward overweight and obese people, even though the prevalence of obesity and being overweight has increased to the point where the majority of the adult population—61 percent—is either overweight or obese.[1] Some groups, such as African American women, have even more startling statistics: 66 percent of us are overweight, and 37 percent are obese.

The negative attitude in society toward the problem of being overweight is manifested in tangible ways. Obese people are more likely to be denied admission into college; they have more trouble renting a residence, and they are less likely to marry than normal weight individuals.[2] Overweight adolescent girls are more likely to have a lower household income and live in poverty once they reach adulthood, compared to normal weight adolescent girls, independent of their baseline socioeconomic status and high school aptitude test scores.[3]

Obesity may limit the opportunity for career advancement; it is also associated with decreased job earnings.[4]

The medical profession is even guilty of harboring misconceptions based on weight. Medical students were found to have an almost uniformly negative reaction to extremely obese people, categorizing them as unpleasant, worthless and bad. The students' attitudes did not change even after they spent some time working with obese patients.[5]

This kind of prejudice and mistreatment can produce deeply rooted feelings of hostility and bitterness— feelings that might seem justified, but are not pleasing to God. One valuable benefit of the spiritual fruit of patience is that it gives us the ability to endure the faults of others. When confronted with negative stereotypes and prejudices, especially those prejudices that result in overt discrimination, a mature level of patience will allow us to "turn the other cheek" (Matt. 5:39). When we are persecuted by intolerant people, it is the forbearance that comes from the Holy Spirit that enables us to forgive those who violate us and pray for those who come against us.

PATIENCE AND TOLERANCE

"Political correctness" was a term coined in the 1990s that refers to how we modify our behavior, our speech and even our thoughts in a way that pleases everyone and offends no one. To that end, the "cripple" of the 1970s was called "handicapped" in the 1980s, and in the politically correct 1990s he was referred to as a "person with disabilities."

The buzzword for political correctness is *tolerance*. Full acceptance of everyone's ideas and lifestyle is required to be considered "tolerant." Anything or anyone deemed intolerant is categorized as politically incorrect. This is why elected officials, who are even remotely interested in reelection, work hard at fine-tuning their air of tolerance.

How do faith and religious belief line up in this "politically correct" paradigm? Interestingly enough, *spirituality* in the broadest sense is considered politically correct. Society has accepted the idea from many world religions that equate spirituality with an open acceptance to all, with no rules to follow and no mandate for repentance or fear of judgment—simply an ethereal connection to the spiritual world or universe.

Tolerance toward sinners

However, Christianity is considered to be politically *in*correct. The Christian faith is perceived by many as a religion filled with endless restrictions and rules. Many non-Christians (and even some Christians) are under the impression that Christianity requires submission to a stringent set of oppressive rules and that anyone who fails to measure up will be rejected. Christians are viewed as intolerant and exclusive to any who do not follow these rules.

Yet Jesus' words reveal that He was willing to include everyone who came to Him, regardless of their status. He said, "Come to me, *all* you who are weary and burdened, and I will give you rest" (Matt. 11:28, emphasis added). Scripture reveals that Jesus made Himself available to anyone and everyone, regardless of who they were, what they did or how they lived. He demonstrated loving tolerance toward sinners.

He placed no restrictions on who was eligible to follow Him, but extended an open invitation to all. Christ epitomized today's idea of political correctness to the extent that His invitation was inclusive for everyone. It became exclusive only by the choice of individuals not to follow Him. Anyone who had a genuine desire to receive Him was totally accepted. The only requirement was to come to Him and accept Him.

We could wonder that since Jesus was open and accepting of everyone, and since His teachings provide the foundation of the Christian faith, why is it that Christianity is perceived as one of the most intolerant of all religions? Part of the problem is the harsh critics who are ignorant of the teachings of Jesus. Another part of the problem is the Christian community that all too often has not treated others in keeping with the loving example of acceptance set by Christ. We as Christians are guilty of being intolerant of *people* rather than being intolerant of *sinfulness*. I believe a chief cause of this misplaced intolerance is the lack of the fruit of the Spirit of patience.

Having addressed our error as Christians of wrongly excluding people because of our intolerance, we must also conclude that people do exclude themselves from the wonderful provisions of Christ when they refuse to come to Him. Relationship with Christ brings wonderful liberty from sin. And it makes possible the development in our lives of His character, including the fruit of patience.

Learning to walk in biblical patience involves endurance and forbearance toward others as well as toward ourselves. These godly traits enable us in our relationship with others to separate individuals from their actions and to love (*agape*) people whom we would otherwise find unlovable. And they allow us to be patient with ourselves while at the same time taking responsibility for our sin.

The very essence of patience in our relationships with others is tolerance; as we grow in grace to be more like Jesus, we are able to be accepting of sinful individuals without ever compromising our stance against sin. Tolerance toward ourselves will allow us to deal with our sin without giving in to an unhealthy attitude of self-loathing while we endure the process of our deliverance.

Intolerance toward sin

Relating to intolerance toward sin, we need to understand the difference between loving the sinner and hating the sin. Jesus accepted sinners; He did not tolerate sin. Anyone who chooses to follow Him must accept His attitude toward their own sin and, through repentance, be delivered from it. This spiritual reality is what makes Christianity politically incorrect according to today's society. Yet intolerance for sin is the first key to being delivered from it.

As the prevalence of obesity has increased among all Americans, including Christians, we have become more and more tolerant of the sins and weaknesses that lead to overeating and that prevent us from a disciplined lifestyle of eating and exercise that would restore health. But this is not the way that Christians are to live. The Bible tells us in Romans 12:2 that we ought not to *conform* to the standards of the world, but we are to be *transformed* through the renewing of our minds.

When our minds are renewed through Christ, then we are transformed; we no longer tolerate those things that do *not* line up with God's commands for living our lives. We begin to understand the true essence of WWJD— What Would Jesus Do? We understand that Jesus would *not* commit the sin of gluttony; He would *not* yield to the desires of the flesh; He would *not* worship food or allow food to control Him (the sin of idolatry); and He would *not* use food to soothe His emotions or numb the sting of past hurts. Most importantly, He would *not* have abused His body—the temple of God—with food. We know that Jesus was fully human and, as such, is a high priest who can fully relate to our humanity (Heb. 4:15). As we choose to allow the Holy Spirit to transform and renew our minds, *we* will take those steps whereby we become more like *Him*.

Patience is one of the beautiful manifestations of Christian love. In the familiar love passage, Paul's first adjective to describe love is *patience*:

> If I speak in the tongues of men and of angels, but have not love, I am only a resounding gong or a clanging cymbal. If I have the gift of prophecy and can fathom all mysteries and all knowledge, and if I have a faith that can move mountains, but have not love, I am nothing. If I give all I possess to the poor and surrender my body to the flames, but have not love, I gain nothing. *Love is patient...*
> —1 CORINTHIANS 13:1–4, EMPHASIS ADDED

As we grow in the Christian faith, our lives should reflect the life of Christ. He was clear in His stance against sin, yet His love and patience toward the poor and outcast drew them to Him. Jesus epitomized patience, but there is no evidence in Scripture that He ever minimized the seriousness of sin. And while we are called to grow in the fruit of the Spirit of patience, which will be manifest in our attitudes of tolerance toward others as well as ourselves, we must never become tolerant of any behavior that is contrary to how the Bible instructs us to live.

Unfortunately, this is often what happens with the

problem of obesity. As we understand our need to be patient with ourselves but intolerant with sin, we can make the right choices that will allow the Holy Spirit to transform the way we think about life, including the place of food and exercise and other health issues.

MY PERSONAL TESTIMONY

Like you, dear reader, I have experienced my own need to grow in the spiritual fruit of patience. I had been in practice for many years before the Lord commissioned me to write this book. And then it took several years for me to complete it. One good reason for the delay was my lack of clinical experience for treating overweight and obese Christians. Another was my need to be mature enough in my own spiritual life to convey effectively the message God had given me. One area of my spiritual life that required personal growth was my lack of patience.

I have never had a weight problem, and I don't have any illnesses that would require me to change my lifestyle. I am aware that this blessing is only by the grace of God. And I don't take the blessing of good health for granted. I strive to maintain my health by eating well, exercising regularly and avoiding those things that would damage my body, like tobacco and excessive alcohol.

God has placed me in a career position where I am required to provide medical care to Christians who *don't* share my values concerning healthy living. Many of my patients *don't* seem to appreciate the blessing of good health. How can I serve them effectively? Only through the fruit of the Spirit of patience.

The fruit of patience is what allows me to connect with all types of people, identify their shortcomings, admonish them to change and expect them to heed my advice—without coming across as condescending or self-righteous. Allowing tolerance and forbearance to "love" my patients through me, I can confront a sensitive issue like obesity, be very candid and direct about the *problem* and not disparage the *person*.

But this was not always my attitude. When I was a new believer I lacked knowledge of the Christian life and had a poor understanding of biblical patience. I must confess, I responded to obese people with the same kind of judgment that the average, normal-weight person does: I couldn't understand what was so difficult about losing weight.

As I grew in godly wisdom, allowing the Holy Spirit to transform my thinking, I also grew in patience. And with the spiritual fruit of patience comes godly compassion. I began to see others in the way God sees them—people precious enough to die for, no matter what their shortcomings.

Biblical patience, or forbearance, also prevents us from imposing our standards on others. When we are patient, we are willing to let others learn of God, grow in the knowledge of Him and take steps toward holy living at their own pace—a pace set by God, not us. This is not to say that we don't encourage others to mature in the faith or that we don't set up systems of accountability for our brothers and sisters who are struggling in a particular area. We ought to provide correction when correction is due, but we do so in a way that is encouraging, not judgmental.

When we lack patience, the faults of others will pre-occupy us to the point that they hinder our ability to serve them. One of my favorite contemporary hymns admonishes us to be like Christ, who, in His amazing grace, "looked beyond my fault and saw my need."[6] The fruit of the Spirit of patience will change our per-spective of others as well as our attitude toward ourselves. First, it allows us to see others through eyes of love as God sees them. Though they may be teeming with error, they are cherished nonetheless. And patience causes us to be introspective so that we don't lose sight of our own defects, those flaws of our past, along with our present imperfections. Humbly, we acknowledge our dependence on the power of God to continue to deliver us from our destruction.

Once I reached greater maturity in the fruit of the Spirit of patience (which the Lord is *still* perfecting in me), I became a better physician to my overweight and obese patients. And the Lord faithfully helped me to complete this manuscript, get the book published and launch the ministry to His precious people with which God has charged me.

Five

The Fruit of the Spirit Is *Kindness...*

If a man shuts his ears to the cry of the poor, he too will cry out and not be answered.

—PROVERBS 21:13

Kindness, the fifth fruit of the Spirit, lies in the heart of the nine fruits. It is at this point—right in the center—that we take a detour from our soul searching and learn how to turn our attention *away* from the subject of body weight.

The most likely reasons that you are reading this book are that you have struggled with obesity or you have a weight-related health problem. So the last thing you may have expected during your reading is to encounter a chapter that ignores your problem. An entire chapter devoted to something other than how to lose weight may not, at first glance, seem to have any merit toward your pursuit of help.

But rest assured that this temporary change in focus does not compromise my objectives. On the contrary, I expect that many will find that the information in this chapter provides what had been the missing link in prior weight loss attempts.

Whenever we're confronted with a challenging or troubling problem, a characteristic response is to become totally absorbed with and immersed in it. It doesn't matter what the problem happens to be— whether it involves our finances, our health or our relationships—this total absorption is typical. We dissect every aspect of the problem and analyze every angle over and over in an attempt to come to terms with the nagging question, "Why me?" It's not long before the problem preoccupies our thoughts throughout the day. And even when we try not to worry, we discover that the problem remains a source of anxiety until the time that it is resolved.

People who have spent years, even decades, struggling with obesity may find that they think about (rather, worry about) some aspect of that struggle on a daily basis. In our discussion about the need to be delivered from the pit of obsession, we focused on the problem of addiction to food. But along with food obsessions, for one struggling with being overweight, there is also the tendency to become obsessed with body weight and appearance. We're all entitled to become a little self-conscious about our weight when we receive the invitation for the high school reunion, but it's a far more serious matter when our weight problem becomes a regular source of anxiety.

In recent years, a number of support groups have been created for obese people. Their goals are to encourage their members to develop a positive attitude about their appearance and to help them overcome this tendency to worry about their weight. There is even a magazine devoted to "full-figure" women. But while some may find support groups and magazines helpful, there is a better way to guard against becoming overly concerned with body weight and physical appearance: the fruit of the Spirit of kindness.

This unlikely secret to your weight loss goals is powerful because demonstrating kindness through acts of service is beneficial not only to the recipient, but also to the giver. As you choose to give the fruit of kindness to others, your life will be enriched immeasurably. My point is best illustrated with a real life example.

Several years ago, my sister developed severe pain throughout her body, along with some other disturbing symptoms. She consulted a number of physicians who ordered a battery of blood tests and a variety of x-rays. All of us were concerned that she might have a disease like lupus or rheumatoid arthritis, but her physical examination and the results of her laboratory tests did not provide us with a specific diagnosis. So ultimately, she was prescribed a number of pain medications and anti-inflammatory drugs without knowing what was wrong with her. To make matters worse, the medications had troubling side effects and barely controlled her pain.

Naturally, she became frustrated with the medical doctors she'd consulted, so she sought the advice of chiropractors, acupuncturists and even a massage therapist. But they too were perplexed. She looked for information at the library and on the Internet without any success. Her symptoms waxed and waned in intensity, but never disappeared. And since she was experiencing them on a daily basis, it didn't take long before she went from simply being concerned and uncomfortable to being totally consumed by her problem. She couldn't understand why she'd been given such a "thorn in the flesh" with which to contend (2 Cor. 12:7).

For some reason, at the height of her frustration, my sister decided to enroll in a hospice training program offered at a nearby hospital, which trained volunteers to assist terminally ill patients and their families. The volunteers were expected to help out with tangible needs such as house cleaning and cooking. But the program was also designed to train them in ways to best serve their patients, walking with them through the dying process. Over time, they were expected to build solid relationships with the patient and family members, such that their presence and words of comfort might ease the pain and help them come to terms with their loss. In short, these volunteers received training in showing kindness.

When my sister began serving dying people in this capacity, a miraculous thing happened. No, her pain didn't go away, but something even more significant occurred. Through sharing with others and demonstrating the fruit of the Spirit of kindness, she was able to put her own problem into perspective. You may be familiar with the saying that poignantly observes, "I cried because I had no shoes, until I met a man who had no feet."[1] When my sister washed the feet—both literally and figuratively—of people with problems far more serious than hers, her own physical problem became more bearable. Though my sister was not challenged by a weight problem, the power of showing kindness will work as dramatically for those who are.

WHY ASK "WHY?"

If there is one thing that distinguishes us from our grandparents, it is that, in general, our grandparents had a higher tolerance for pain. Our standard of living and our quality of life have improved dramatically in only a few generations. The life expectancy has increased because we are able to treat diseases that were once uniformly fatal. It is now a rare tragedy for a woman to die in childbirth, for example, though this was once a not uncommon outcome.

And it hasn't been too long ago that people spent many years of their life working in places that were physically unsafe or that exposed them to toxic chemicals. But while our grandparents endured great trials, they were not as inclined as we are today to seek an explanation for their pain. Simply put, suffering was just a part of life.

Today, however, our living standards are more comfortable, and as a result, our tolerance for pain is much lower. Along with that low pain threshold, philosophies of today have developed in us an inordinate need to know why. "Why did God allow this to happen?" "Why, if He loves me, would He subject me to this?" "Why me, when I've tried to do right all of my life?" Suffering is no longer accepted as a part of life; it is seen as an exceptional circumstance for which we deserve an explanation.

The New Age "me"

How did this happen? How is it that trials that would have been handled in stride by our grandparents shake us to the foundation of our souls? Why do we become so frustrated and angry when faced with a difficult life situation? I've concluded the answer is attributable in part to the prevalent New Age philosophy of today that encourages the aggrandizement of self.

One common thread in New Age doctrine is the exaltation of mankind. Some of the teaching equates man's nature with the divine nature of God. It goes a step beyond the Christian doctrine, which says that the Spirit of God abides in a follower of Christ and asserts that man himself is divine. The essence of the teaching lies in its message that is one of self-centeredness—my needs, my issues, my good, along with the ever-present quest for my inner man. Consequently, when faced with a challenge, the person who follows New Age theology—consciously or unconsciously—feels entitled to an explanation.

Though self-centeredness is at the core of New Age theology, self-centeredness is not Christian doctrine. Rather, a Christian lifestyle presumes that we *refrain* from selfish thinking and selfish behavior. The apostle Paul warned believers, "Do not think of yourself more highly than you ought, but rather think of yourself with sober judgment, in accordance with the measure of faith God has given you" (Rom. 12:3). He goes on to say that believers must learn to "honor one another above yourselves" (v. 10).

The Bible never says that believers will be exempt from suffering, but it *does* encourage us to guard against becoming overwhelmed by our circumstances. As Christians, we are to *expect* trials and, when they come, to *endure* them and *grow* from the experience. James gave believers this valuable perspective regarding trials:

> Consider it pure joy, my brothers, whenever you face trials of many kinds, because you know that the testing of your faith develops perseverance. Perseverance must finish its work so that you may be mature and complete, not lacking anything.
>
> —JAMES 1:2–4

And Peter taught believers to:

> Make every effort to add to your faith goodness; and to goodness, knowledge; and to knowledge, self-control; and to self-control, perseverance; and to perseverance, godliness; and to godliness, brotherly kindness; and to brotherly kindness, love.
>
> —2 PETER 1:5–7

The fruit of the Spirit of kindness is that special fruit we demonstrate to others as "brotherly kindness." Focusing on serving others gives us a wonderful perspective and helps us to handle our trials in a manner that is Christlike. When kindness is richly manifested in us, it gives us the power to exchange our question of "Why me, Lord?" for a humble "Thank You, Lord." The problems of obesity and being overweight have the propensity to cause our focus to be self-centered. Showing kindness to others helps to protect us against this defeating self-absorption.

SUFFICIENT GRACE

I am not suggesting that we should never, under any

circumstance, ask God, "Why me?" All throughout the Scriptures, we find that men and women subjected to adversity did just that. Job was a righteous man, so righteous that even God said, "There is no one on earth like him; he is blameless and upright, a man who fears God and shuns evil" (Job 1:8). But when tragedy struck, Job wanted an explanation.

When the prophet Jeremiah was beaten and put into the stocks for proclaiming God's message, he complained to God that he had received nothing but persecution and sorrow in return for his faithfulness (Jer. 20).

And I imagine that even Joseph, while sitting in prison, innocent of the charges that placed him there, had to wonder every now and then about God's purpose for his suffering. These are just a few examples of men and women of the Bible who suffered and wanted to know the reason why. But if there is one thing we should learn from their experiences, it's that we shouldn't spend too much time seeking an explanation for our pain.

When we feel entitled to an explanation for our difficult circumstances, we run the risk of compromising our reverence for God by doubting His omniscience. We can get so absorbed with our problem—especially problems that are related to our health—that we forget that God is all knowing and always in control. We must diligently guard ourselves against becoming completely engrossed in trying to figure out our circumstances.

From the apostle Paul we learn a valuable lesson about facing trials. He was faced with a challenge that he referred to as a thorn in his flesh:

> To keep me from becoming conceited because of these surpassingly great revelations, there was given me a thorn in my flesh, a messenger of Satan, to torment me. Three times I pleaded with the Lord to take it away from me. But he said to me, "My grace is sufficient for you, for my power is made perfect in weakness." Therefore I will boast all the more gladly about my weaknesses, so that Christ's power may rest on me. That is why, for Christ's sake, I delight in weaknesses, in insults, in hardships, in persecutions, in difficulties. For when I am weak, then I am strong.
>
> —2 CORINTHIANS 12:7–10

When he was afflicted with this problem, Paul didn't hesitate to pray that God would take it away. We don't know the nature of the problem, but whatever it was, it troubled Paul enough that he asked on more than one occasion that God would remove it. Eventually, however, it became clear that God had no intentions of doing so.

Please indulge me, for the sake of discussion, and let's imagine that the thorn in Paul's flesh was obesity. How might Paul have responded? He might have challenged God, demanding to know why it was so difficult for him to lose weight. He could have asked, "Why me, Lord? After all the things that I've done in Your name and all the time I've spent serving You, why won't You answer my prayer and take these pounds away?"

Paul could have spent hours thinking about how wonderful life would be if he didn't weigh so much. Then he might spend even more hours reflecting on all the mistakes he had made in the past, wondering if his weight problem was some form of retribution. ("If I hadn't persecuted all those Christians, would God have allowed me to become so fat?")

Paul might have become so self-absorbed that he spent most of his day counting calories, checking his weight and measuring his waistline. He might have stood in the mirror to examine himself each morning, only to reflect sadly on that image all day long. He could have wallowed in self-pity and become so self-conscious about his clothing size that he refused to travel on any more missionary journeys until he lost twenty pounds.

Whatever Paul's thorn in the flesh was, he could have responded to it in a selfish way, becoming totally absorbed with his circumstances. He could have worried about his problem to the point that he was ineffective in spreading the gospel. After all, he couldn't very well speak about the Good News of Christ if in his heart he felt slighted by the Lord or was bitter about his condition.

Had Paul responded in any of these hypothetical ways, he would have missed an opportunity for tremendous spiritual growth. But he knew that having a right relationship with God did not exempt him from trouble. Remember that it was Paul who admonished believers not to think more highly of themselves than they ought (Rom. 12:3).

He refused to let his thorn in the flesh, no matter how distressing, give him a reason to wallow in self-pity. Instead, Paul received the promise of the Master who declared, "My grace is sufficient for you, for my power is made perfect in weakness" (2 Cor. 12:9).

Paul's bold response was, "Therefore I will boast all the more gladly about my weaknesses, so that Christ's power may rest on me...For when I am weak, then I am strong" (vv. 9–10). He understood real dependency on the power of God to overcome his weaknesses.

We should strive to respond to adversity the way that Paul did. He turned his attention off of his problem and on to Christ. When it became obvious that the thorn in his flesh was something he would have to live with, the lesson he learned was that the grace of God was sufficient for him in any circumstance. He didn't allow himself to spend too much time focusing on the negative aspects of his condition. Instead, he grew in the knowledge that the grace of God was all he needed, and that is what made his weakness a source of strength.

A classic old hymn expresses this dependency this way:

> I am weak but Thou art strong;
> Jesus, keep me from all wrong;
> I'll be satisfied as long
> As I walk, let me walk close to Thee.
> Just a closer walk with Thee,
> Grant it, Jesus, is my plea,
> Daily walking close to Thee,
> Let it be, dear Lord, let it be.[2]

Our strongest desire has to be a closer walk with God and a coming to the full knowledge that His grace is sufficient, no matter what our circumstances.

How does the spiritual fruit of kindness relate to God's sufficient grace? According to Scripture, God's grace is manifested through the fresh kindness He pours out upon us each day:

Because of the LORD'S great love we are not consumed, for his compassions never fail. They are
new every morning; great is your faithfulness.
                              —LAMENTATIONS 3:22–23

For his merciful kindness is great toward us: and
the truth of the LORD endureth for ever. Praise ye
the LORD.
                                   —PSALM 117:2, KJV

Paul's lesson learned from his thorn in the flesh—
and our lesson for difficult situations, including
obesity—is that the grace of God is adequate, no matter
what our condition. His kindness toward us is so profound that it makes our pain pale in comparison.
When we begin to view our situation from the perspective of God's mercy, it will help us realize that whatever
the problem happens to be, it's like a tiny grain of sand,
almost imperceptible, on the endless glistening
seashores of the Lord's kindness.

And this same kindness dwells in the believer
through the power of the Holy Spirit. As we yield to
Him in cultivating and expressing kindness, we render
on earth the kindness that God imparts to us from
heaven. We then emulate for others that which God has
done for us. In this respect, kindness becomes thera-
peutic: It liberates us from the burden of our
circumstance, placing our trouble in proper perspective.

Expressing kindness is so vital to Christian life, that
in Matthew 25, Jesus equates serving those in need to
serving Him.

It is my desire that every person reading this book
will be able to apply these principles toward reaching a

healthier weight. But I'm wise enough to know that many will not, and for them, obesity will remain a thorn in the flesh. If you happen to fall into this category, then you have a choice to make: You can spend your days disappointed by your weight, or you can grow in the knowledge of God's grace, understanding that it is sufficient in any circumstance. The fruit of the Spirit of kindness will help you make the right choice.

Six

The Fruit of
the Spirit Is
Goodness...

Keep falsehood and lies far from me;
give me neither poverty nor riches, but
give me only my daily bread.
—PROVERBS 30:8

When I first thought about writing this book, I discussed it with my husband, and after a period of fasting and prayer, we felt confident that this was one of the ways that God would have me use the gifts and talents He had given me. We felt the book would provide a foundation of biblical principles that would inspire the reader to believe God for deliverance from weight-related problems.

During my research of the topic, I studied the word *diet*. You may realize that *diet* can be used as a noun or a verb. The noun, in *Webster's Ninth New Collegiate Dictionary*, is defined as "food and drink regularly provided or consumed; habitual nourishment." Our frame of reference is to spiritual food—the fruit of the Spirit. When these principles govern our lives as believers, we walk in liberty from sin. Our lives are richer when we "regularly consume" and "habitually nourish" ourselves by pursuing the things of God.

As a verb, *diet* means "to eat sparingly or according to prescribed rules." We do not recommend that you live life trying to eat sparingly or according to prescribed rules. Losing weight does not require us to become slaves to food, and this is exactly what happens when we try to apply a strict set of rules to something as normal and natural as eating.

For our purposes in this book, when we refer to natural food, the word *diet* is a noun and not a verb—that is, habitual nourishment. We don't want to be culinary prisoners; we want to be free to nourish our bodies with a wide selection of foods and learn to supply them with just the right amount—not too much, not too little. The problem is that too many people have trouble in determining what is the right amount. When the words *not too much* are easier said than done, we find ourselves faced with obesity, being overweight and weight-related health problems.

We will discuss the "not-too-much" problem in a later chapter. As we turn our discussion now to the spiritual fruit of goodness, we want to consider the goodness of God to provide for us all the nourishment we need for health and well-being of body, mind and spirit.

THE PROVISIONS OF GOD

If I were asked to list the many ways that God manifests His love and mercy toward us, meeting our nutritional needs would be placed near the top. Psalm 136 is a beautiful psalm of thanksgiving for God's enduring love. It begins with an acknowledgment of God as the creator of the universe (verses 1–9), then speaks of Him as the one who is able to deliver us from the hand of our enemies (verses 10–22), and concludes in recognition of His provisions:

> To the One who remembered us in our low estate
>   His love endures forever.
> And freed us from our enemies,
>   His love endures forever.
> And who gives food to every creature.
>   His love endures forever.
> Give thanks to the God of heaven.
>   His love endures forever.
>
> —PSALM 136:23–26

One of the names of God is *Jehovah-Jireh*. Its Hebrew meaning reflects the generous attribute of God as a loving provider. In Genesis 22, God tested Abraham by calling him to sacrifice his son Isaac. Abraham obeyed God by taking Isaac to the mountain, binding him to the altar and even lifting the knife to slay him. Just as he was prepared to bring the knife down on his son, God stopped him and provided an animal for him to sacrifice instead:

> Abraham looked up and there in a thicket he saw a ram caught by its horns. He went over and took the ram and sacrificed it as a burnt offering instead of his son. So Abraham called that place The LORD Will Provide.
>
> —GENESIS 22:13–14

Abraham learned to know the goodness of God in a new way that day as a faithful provider to those who obey His commands. In Psalm 37, David declared the goodness of God as well:

> I was young and now I am old, yet I have never
> seen the righteous forsaken or their children beg-
> ging bread.
>
> —PSALM 37:25

Even Jesus, in the model prayer He taught His disciples, included the appeal to "give us today our daily
bread" (Matt. 6:11). When we pray in this way, we are
acknowledging that it is God in His goodness, and God
alone, who provides for us and sustains us. We trust
Him each day to supply us with the things we need to
survive, and we admit that we are incapable of meeting
those needs by ourselves.

From the beginning of creation, God has consistently
shown Himself to be the One who provides for us and
meets our every need, including our need for food.
During the years that the Israelites spent wandering in
the wilderness, their nutritional needs were met with
manna, a divine food that came from out of the
heavens. And while God is still able to provide us with
miracle food from the skies, our source of food is the
richness of God's good earth.

THE BOUNTIFUL EARTH

The earth is the source of our clothing, our shelter and,
of course, our food. God, "who richly provides us with
everything for our enjoyment" (1 Tim. 6:17), has made
the earth produce a bounty of foods in a wide variety of
tastes and textures not just for our sustenance, but also
for our enjoyment.

Our flesh requires food to survive. There is nothing
wrong with enjoying the act of eating and the fellowship

that comes with breaking bread together. There should be a healthy balance between sustenance for survival and enjoyment of eating. Unfortunately, there is a tendency to allow the pendulum to swing too far in the direction of enjoyment or too far toward survival alone. At one extreme we find excess, indulgence and gluttony; at the other there is little enjoyment in eating because of unwarranted restraint and feelings of guilt.

As we express the spiritual fruit of goodness, we celebrate food as a blessing from God—a gift to us from Jehovah-Jireh. Food should never assume a more significant role than what God intended. It is not an idol to be worshiped, a friend to the lonely, a stress-reducing agent or an antidepressant. We turn to God, the source and supplier of the gift of food, and we worship Him—not His provisions. We seek His face in times of trouble. We look to Him—not our plate—in times of stress. And we look to Him—not the refrigerator—when we are depressed or lonely. We keep the gift and the Giver separate and distinct, learning to give thanks to God for providing us with food to enjoy, never permitting that food to fulfill any need beyond which it was intended.

Nourishment and enjoyment are the two main purposes for which food was created. The gift of food is supplied through plants and animals. During the 1950s science categorized food into four major groups—the meat group, the milk group, the bread and cereal group and the fruit and vegetable group. This "basic four" concept helped with meal planning and served to remind us of the importance of eating a variety of foods. But by the 1990s, as our knowledge of

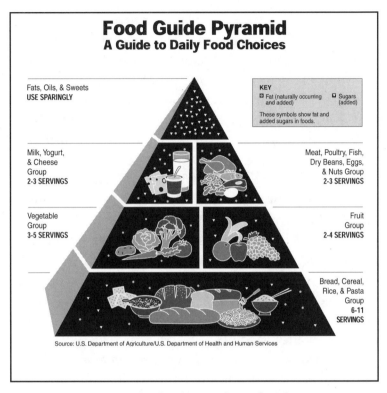

nutrition increased, the basic four food groups were replaced with a pyramid.

The pyramid is made up of five food groups. A well-balanced diet contains foods from each of these five categories in serving sizes that are proportional to the area in the pyramid represented by that particular type of food. The pyramid's three lower tiers are comprised of the nutrient-rich foods that provide us with everything needed to sustain life. The top of the pyramid is represented by foods that consist primarily of fat and sugar. These foods have a low nutritional value and are the main source of "empty calories"—calories that provide few, if any, nutrients.

Along with eating the correct proportion of food from the different groups, it is also important to broaden our selection of foods from within each category. Different foods are rich in different nutrients. A diet that includes a wide variety of foods is not only appealing to our taste buds, but it will also provide us with an adequate supply of the vitamins and nutrients essential to good health.

Once while grocery shopping with my daughter Grace, I was looking over the asparagus when a woman standing nearby smiled at my daughter and told her that she had never tried asparagus. She was curious to know whether or not Grace liked it. The woman was at least fifty years old. Grace, who at the ripe age of six had eaten asparagus fairly regularly, seemed a bit amazed that a woman her age had never tried it and told her that it tasted OK.

While this woman may have eaten vegetables every day, because her selection was limited, her diet may not have provided the recommended amounts of certain vitamins and nutrients. Asparagus is not just a tasty vegetable; it supplies us with vitamin E, one of the antioxidant vitamins that work to protect our cells from damage.

The shape of the food pyramid—large at the base and small at the apex—is a visual reminder that serves to help us to follow a healthy diet. Grains, cereals and breads are found in the base. These kinds of foods are the staple of a well-balanced diet and should be consumed in larger quantities than the other groups. The apex is the smallest part of the pyramid and is represented by foods that ought to be eaten sparingly.

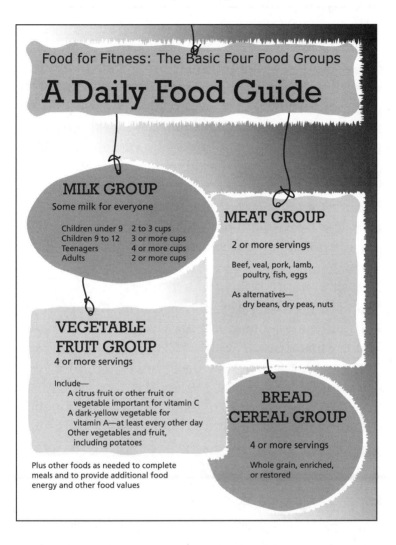

Food for Fitness: The Basic Four Food Groups

A Daily Food Guide

MILK GROUP

Some milk for everyone

Children under 9	2 to 3 cups
Children 9 to 12	3 or more cups
Teenagers	4 or more cups
Adults	2 or more cups

MEAT GROUP

2 or more servings

Beef, veal, pork, lamb,
poultry, fish, eggs

As alternatives—
dry beans, dry peas, nuts

VEGETABLE FRUIT GROUP

4 or more servings

Include—
A citrus fruit or other fruit or
vegetable important for vitamin C
A dark-yellow vegetable for
vitamin A—at least every other day
Other vegetables and fruit,
including potatoes

Plus other foods as needed to complete
meals and to provide additional food
energy and other food values

BREAD CEREAL GROUP

4 or more servings

Whole grain, enriched,
or restored

Unlike the pyramid, the "basic four" food groups were represented by a chart that visually depicted an equal area for each food group. This symbol gave the impression that a balanced diet consisted of equal representation from each of the four food groups. A "healthy" meal, then, could have as large a serving of meat as it did grains and bread, or fruits and vegetables.

Until only recently, it was unheard of to prepare a meal, especially dinner, that did not include meat. When I was growing up, meat was the focal point of the plate—everything else was called a "side dish." Vegetarianism seemed like a radical and "un-American" practice. Over the past four decades our understanding of food and nutrition has increased dramatically. We understand that we need more of some foods and less of others for a balanced diet. Despite this new knowledge, the belief that the different food groups deserve equal representation is still ingrained in many people's minds.

Several years ago, my mother came by to visit just as I was serving lunch to Grace, who was three years old at the time. On her plate was a serving of couscous, along with broccoli with cheese. She had a glass of milk to drink. My mother, who in years past was a diligent follower of the basic four food groups, was by this time fairly knowledgeable about the latest information regarding food and nutrition. But in spite of this new knowledge, she still expressed some pretty strong reservations about serving a "growing child" a meatless meal. Old habits—especially those related to food—are hard to die.

But even though old habits tend to stick with us, as Christians, we are called to follow the leading of the Holy Spirit and not live by any hard-to-break regimen. Every aspect of our lives, including what we eat and how we eat it, should be grounded in godly wisdom. We are regularly discovering more facts about the impact our diets have on our health. As we learn about the links between diet and disease, we must accept that old habits regarding food—if they're bad habits—need changing. As we choose to change, we can draw upon the power of the Holy Spirit to help us in implementing that change.

"IS THIS OK TO EAT?"

God in His goodness has ordained that the earth produce food for us. He only requires that we receive the gift of food in moderation so that we can enjoy health. Having a solid understanding of the way we ought to eat does not require an advanced degree in biochemistry or physiology. If we start by using godly wisdom—wisdom in the form of common sense—and simply examine the "fearful and wonderful" way that God has created us, we can get some understanding of what types of foods are most appropriate for us without taking a course in clinical nutrition.

Since eating starts in the mouth, it makes sense to examine the fearful and wonderful way that God created our teeth. Humans have relatively few sharp teeth—we have more flat molars than we do pointy canines. God created us with a predominance of flat teeth that are useful for grinding, with fewer sharp teeth that are needed for tearing meat. Unlike the carnivorous lions and tigers, whose teeth are ideally suited for ripping into flesh, most of our teeth are designed for grinding plants—grains, legumes, fruits and vegetables.

It should come as no surprise, then, to find that our bowel habits are more regular when we consume a diet that contains a large amount of high-fiber, plant-derived foods, with a comparatively smaller amount of meat. Constipation is rarely a problem for people who eat plenty of fruits, vegetables, legumes and whole grains. But the benefits of a high-fiber diet extend beyond bowel regularity.

It has been shown that diets with a low fiber content increase the risk of type 2 diabetes in adults,[1] and that increasing the intake of dietary fiber (especially soluble fiber) above the level currently recommended by the American Diabetic Association will improve the blood sugar control and reduce the cholesterol and triglyceride levels in patients with type 2 diabetes.[2] And since God created us with teeth that are better equipped for these types of foods, we shouldn't be surprised to learn that diet-related illnesses are more common in people who eat an excessive amount of meat relative to plant-derived foods.

Godly wisdom requires that we restrict our diets to foods that generate health. But this is nothing new— dietary restrictions have been in place since Adam and Eve lived in the Garden of Eden. Rather than consider this restriction as a form of punishment or deprivation, we need to understand that in God's goodness, it is His intent to protect us from harm.

Before the Fall of man, God instructed Adam that mankind and animals were to live off the plants of the earth:

> Then God said, "I give you every seed-bearing plant on the face of the whole earth and every tree that has fruit with seed in it. They will be yours for food. And to all the beasts of the earth and all the birds of the air and all the creatures that move on

the ground—everything that has the breath of life
in it—I give every green plant for food." And it
was so.

—GENESIS 1:29–30

Man and beast ate freely from every plant in the
garden, including the fruit of the tree of life, which gave
eternal life (Gen. 3:22). So prior to the Fall, neither
man nor animal experienced death. As such, even the
very concept of killing for the purpose of food was
nonexistent since animals experienced eternal life just
as man did.

The diet in the Garden of Eden was in keeping with
this state of eternal life—there were no carnivores
because there was no bloodshed. Vegetarianism was the
first diet prescribed by God. There is nothing wrong
with practicing vegetarianism. A vegetarian diet can
provide all the nutrients required for life. But we
mustn't assume that it is somehow a "better" way to eat
simply because it was the first diet prescribed by God.
Even angels eat meat (c.f., Gen. 18:1–8). The reason
man's original diet was comprised exclusively of plants
was because, prior to the Fall of man, there was no
death through bloodshed for man or for beasts.

With the Fall of man came death, destruction and
the shedding of blood. God Himself, after confronting
Adam and Eve about their sin, slaughtered an animal in
order to provide them with clothing (Gen. 3:21). The
original condition of man—specifically man's relationship to the animal world—was altered. Animal skin
became acceptable for clothing and animal flesh for
food. This is documented later in the Book of Genesis
with the story of the great flood and the covenant that

God established with Noah after the flood. The waters receded, Noah and his family exited the ark into a brand-new world, and God immediately blessed them and established a covenant:

> Be fruitful and increase in number and fill the earth. The fear and dread of you will fall upon all the beasts of the earth and all the birds of the air, upon every creature that moves along the ground, and upon all the fish of the sea; they are given into your hands. Everything that lives and moves will be food for you. Just as I gave you the green plants, I now give you everything.
> —GENESIS 9:1–3

The circumstances for both man and beast had changed. The relationship of animal to man was now grounded in fear. While man was expected to treat animals humanely, he was nevertheless permitted to kill them for food and clothing. The human diet changed from being exclusively vegetarian to carnivorous. Keep in mind that God permitted animals to be used as a source of food as part of a covenant of *blessing* to man—eating meat is not "wrong."

A carnivorous diet does, however, require that we exercise more care and follow certain precautions to avoid consuming harmful bacteria and parasites. Unlike fruits and vegetables, which can be eaten raw (and are usually better in their raw state), undercooked or contaminated red meat, poultry and fish can lead to a variety of illnesses, some even life-threatening. This can be avoided by using fresh products from quality sources, keeping your hands and preparation area clean and cooking the meat thoroughly.

Noah's three sons and their wives began the process of repopulating the earth, and from these three families descended all the races of mankind. The Hebrew people are descendants of Noah's son Shem; they would be called by God to live under the rules and regulations known as the Mosaic Law. The Law included guidelines for every aspect of living, including extensive instruction on diet. There were rules concerning what to eat, when to eat it and how to prepare it. It is important for us to understand the purpose of the Mosaic Law and why these restrictions were placed upon the Hebrews so that we avoid any confusion regarding God's dietary laws.

The Mosaic Law was implemented for the purpose of separation, preservation and revelation. The Jews were to remain separate as a race and not intermingle with other people because Jesus, the Messiah, was to be born of them. The Law served to preserve this race because all of its restrictions were beneficial: They promoted health, they limited the spread of disease, and they served to maintain justice and civil order among the people. Finally, the Mosaic Law was able to reveal the sinfulness of man and provide proof that man was incapable of following all of the precepts of a holy God. It revealed beyond a doubt that we needed a Savior who would pay the price for our many violations of His law.

Jesus came to fulfill the Mosaic Law so that every man who believed in Him would no longer be held accountable to the Law. We now live in a state of grace through faith in Jesus Christ and are no longer bound by legalism. Despite this liberty, far too many Christians are legalistic about their diets. For example, some Christians adamantly refuse to eat pork, not because they dislike the taste or because they have a health problem that would require them to limit or omit pork from their diets (e.g., high cholesterol). They choose to completely eliminate it from the menu simply because pork has a "bad reputation." They cited the fact that it was one of the many foods that the Mosaic Law specifically excluded from the Hebrew diet.

Don't misunderstand me—there is nothing wrong with controlling our appetites and limiting (or even eliminating) certain foods from our diets. By doing this, we keep our "flesh" under subjection, and we are then better equipped to handle sinful desires when they surface in other areas of our lives. But while some level of dietary restraint is necessary and beneficial, too often we subject ourselves to unreasonable and unnecessary dietary restrictions. We mistakenly think that our self-imposed constraints will win us brownie points in the sight of God, forgetting that He has already paid a tremendous price for our liberty.

When dietary restrictions are implemented because of legalism, there is a significant risk that the restrictions will become a catalyst for self-righteousness. I regularly encounter Christians who brag about their "good" eating habits. To make matters worse, they are often pretty judgmental toward people who don't follow the same dietary rules. Jesus had a lot to say about the sin of self-righteousness. On one occasion He described two men who were praying in the temple, one a Pharisee and the other a tax collector:

> Two men went up to the temple to pray, one a
> Pharisee and the other a tax collector. The
> Pharisee stood up and prayed about himself:
> "God, I thank you that I am not like the other
> men—robbers, evildoers, adulterers—or even like
> this tax collector. I fast twice a week and give a
> tenth of all I get."
>
> But the tax collector stood at a distance. He
> would not even look up to heaven, but beat his
> breast and said, "God, have mercy on me, a sinner."
> —LUKE 18:10–13

The Bible says that Jesus was speaking to "some who
were confident of their own righteousness and looked
down on everybody else" (Luke 18:9). When we
become legalistic about our diets, we run the same risk
of being confident in our own self-righteousness. Allow
me to suggest the following parody of this same
parable that results when we become self-righteous in
our approach to diet:

> Two men went up to the temple to pray, one a
> physically fit vegetarian and the other a grossly
> overweight carnivore. The vegetarian stood up and
> prayed about himself: "God, I thank you that I am
> not like other men—beef eaters, pork eaters, egg
> eaters—or even like this fat man here. I fast twice a
> week, and each day I eat ten servings of fruits and
> vegetables."
>
> But the obese man stood at a distance. He
> would not even look up to heaven, but beat his
> thick chest and prayed sincerely, "God, have mercy
> on me, a glutton."

No acceptable or unacceptable foods

God's covenant with Noah, combined with the blessing of grace and the fulfillment of the Mosaic Law through Christ, makes it clear that there are no "acceptable" and "unacceptable" foods, but that God has created the earth to produce a variety of foods for our nourishment and enjoyment.

All food should be eaten in moderation, and some foods should be limited or even eliminated from the diet for medical reasons or for weight loss purposes. This does not make the food "bad"; it simply means that it is not beneficial for selected individuals with specific problems. There may even come a time when those foods that were once eliminated from the diet are no longer completely off-limits but only need to be handled with a greater degree of self-control.

As believers, we need to pray and seek godly counsel for wisdom in determining which foods are appropriate, given our particular situations, and we need to ask God for the power to control our tendency to indulge ourselves. It was Jesus who said, "Listen and understand. What goes into a man's mouth does not make him 'unclean,' but what comes out of his mouth, that is what makes him 'unclean'" (Matt. 15:10–11). What comes out of our mouths reflects what's inside of our hearts. If the goodness of God dwells there, we will be able to make right choices regarding how to nourish His temple. And we will enjoy the variety of foods, in moderation, that He has given to us in the wonderful provision of Jehovah-Jireh.

Seven

The Fruit of the Spirit Is *Faithfulness...*

Many a man claims to have unfailing love, but a faithful man who can find?
—PROVERBS 20:6

This proverb, written hundreds of years ago by the one of the world's wisest men, can be paraphrased in simple terms for the twenty-first century to read, "Talk is cheap." It's easy to make a declaration or to vow a vow, but living up to that declaration or vow is an entirely different matter. The high rate of divorce gives us evidence of this truth. Men and women who claim their unfailing love—not just to each other but in the presence of witnesses, and not just as small talk but in the form of a vow—are found heading for divorce court when the going gets tough.

If we fail to cultivate the fruit of faithfulness in our lives, we are doomed to fail in our relationship with God, our relationships with others and even our relationship with ourselves. As we allow the Holy Spirit to work in our hearts, helping us to cultivate this fruit, we will begin to understand the secret of faithfulness to a blessed life. Because faithfulness is closely related to faith, we need to understand the dynamic of faith in God and the difficulty that doubt presents to cultivating faithfulness in our lives.

DEALING WITH DOUBT

The eleventh chapter of the Book of Hebrews opens with a profound truth: "Now faith is the substance of things hoped for, the evidence of things not seen" (v. 1, KJV). Belief in God is only possible through faith. God is not someone we see with our natural eyes, but through faith, we have solid evidence of His existence. Believing in God requires faith, and believing in what God is able to do requires a double dose of faith—first, to believe that He exists, and second, to believe that He is able to work in the lives of His people.

Somewhere between the faith to believe in God and the faith required to believe that God is able we find a quagmire of doubt. In that deadly quagmire many people are losing the weight loss battle. They believe that God exists, but they cannot be sure that He is able to help them in their personal struggles.

Anyone who has ever weight cycled knows that with each new attempt to lose weight, the measure of self-doubt increases. That doubt is fueled by past failures. Each pound and every ounce that return serve to strengthen the uncertainty. It's then only a matter of time before self-doubt and doubt of God's ability to help is strong enough to thwart any fresh attempts to lose weight.

People in the weight loss industry know that doubt is a formidable force. To counteract its power, they tantalize potential customers with promises that are nothing short of being too good to be true. So we muster up the confidence to try one more plan, only because the "Before and After" testimonial photographs are incredible enough to release us from doubt's grip for the moment.

Doubt is an issue common to every person. The issue is not a question of *whether* we will feel doubt; it is a question of how to handle doubt *when* it comes. The Bible gives many examples of men and women who experienced doubt. When the Lord told Moses that He would provide meat for the Israelites to eat in the wilderness, Moses responded by saying:

> Here I am among six hundred thousand men on foot, and you say, "I will give them meat to eat for a whole month!" Would they have enough if flocks and herds were slaughtered for them? Would they have enough if all the fish in the sea were caught for them?
>
> —NUMBERS 11:21–22

The apostle Thomas, whom many have dubbed *doubting* Thomas, wanted tangible proof of the resurrection of Christ before he would believe. He told his fellow disciples, "Unless I see the nail marks in his hands and put my finger where the nails were, and put my hand into his side, I will not believe it" (John 20:25). And John the Baptist sent his followers to ask Christ, "Are you the one who was to come, or shall we expect someone else?" (Matt. 11:3). One of the more poignant passages from the Bible is the account of the man whose son was possessed by a mute spirit. This desperate father cried out to Christ, "I do believe; help me overcome my unbelief!" (Mark 9:24).

In all four of these examples, doubt arises partly because these very ordinary people were facing a discouraging set of circumstances. God called Moses to lead the Israelites out of slavery in Egypt. The people witnessed the miraculous hand of God move on their behalf in order to set them free after centuries of living in bondage. But despite this blessing, they became discontent and turned their backs on God once they were delivered. Moses was burdened and discouraged by their constant complaining.

For Thomas, it seemed that all hope in the coming Messiah died with the crucifixion of Jesus. He had devoted three years to following Christ and learning of Him. His loyalty to Jesus was evident in his willingness to die for him (John 11:16). But when his hope was challenged, Thomas became overwhelmed with doubt.

> *Disappointment or discouragement can cause feelings of doubt in the most mature believers.*

John the Baptist had preached in the wilderness of the coming of Christ and how vitally important it was for everyone to prepare themselves for the Messiah. But soon after meeting Jesus, baptizing Jesus and proclaiming to his followers, "Look, the Lamb of God, who takes away the sin of the world!" (John 1:29), he found himself alone and wrongfully imprisoned.

And finally, the father of the mute son, like many of the people Christ healed, had lived with his son's condition for years—in this case, for all of the child's life. He had certainly sought medical attention many times throughout the years, and undoubtedly he felt periods of hope after being prescribed a new form of treatment or a new medication. But the illness continued to plague his son, and every recurring seizure brought with it the sting of disappointment.

Disappointment or discouragement can cause feelings of doubt in the most mature believers. Certainly if John the Baptist, who was aware of the presence of Christ while he was yet in his mother's womb, could feel a twinge of doubt, then we should not be surprised when we feel it. For many who struggle with being overweight, the disappointment and discouragement that comes with a failed diet plan or regained weight sets the stage for doubt.

The wrong way

What, then, is the best way to handle doubt? First, let's look at the wrong way. Doubt becomes a problem when it is not acknowledged for what it is. From the time a person becomes a Christian, he or she is instructed in the importance of faith. Faith is necessary in prayer, in evangelism and in worship; according to Hebrews 11:6, it is even necessary in order to please God: "And without faith it is impossible to please God." So when feelings of doubt arise, there is the tendency to ignore them or suppress them, because to acknowledge them would be tantamount to acknowledging weak faith. The reasoning goes something like this:

> I feel doubt; *therefore,*
> my faith must be weak; *therefore,*
> my profession that I am Christian—a claim that
> requires faith—is challenged.

If we apply this same reasoning to weight loss, it might sound something like this:

> I've been unsuccessful with countless weight loss plans; *therefore,*
> I doubt I will ever be able to lose weight and keep it off; *therefore,*
> I must not have faith that God is able to help me in this struggle.

The last thought is too difficult to entertain, so instead, the obesity is accepted and doubt is suppressed. This suppression is done either consciously or subconsciously, but in either case, the result is the same—through accepting that which is unacceptable, the person's faith does not seem to be challenged. The reasoning then becomes:

> I have been unsuccessful with countless weight loss plans, and
> I have doubt that I will ever lose weight; *therefore,*
> I choose to stay overweight.

The right way

The biggest tragedy to this line of reasoning is the false notion that feelings of doubt are indicative of an absence of faith. They are not. Doubt only signifies that faith is being challenged. John the Baptist was a man of strong faith, but when circumstances challenged his faith (the circumstance of being imprisoned for speaking the truth), then doubt surfaced. Rather than hide his doubt or ignore it, he took it to the only one who could ease it—Jesus Christ. And his honesty was not met with a rebuke but with words of assurance and encouragement from the Lord:

> Go back and report to John what you have seen
> and heard: The blind receive sight, the lame walk,
> those who have leprosy are cured, the deaf hear,
> the dead are raised, and the good news is
> preached to the poor. Blessed is the man who
> does not fall away on account of me.
> —LUKE 7:22–23

Instead of suppressing our doubt, we need to take it
to the Lord. There we will be encouraged also that the
Lord is able to get involved in our situations. The discouragement and disappointment of weight regain
and weight cycling can cause doubt. If you have been
discouraged to the point that you have resolved to
never again tackle your weight problem, you need to
separate your faith from your feelings of doubt. In this
case, doubt is nothing more than an emotion produced from feelings of inadequacy or fear of failure.
Our faith, on the other hand, reflects our belief in God
and our knowledge that He is able to do "immeasurably more than all we ask or imagine" (Eph. 3:20). We
aren't governed by our emotions, but by our faith.

If past failures have been a negative influence on your
resolve, then model your response after the man with
the mute son. First, accept the fact that the problem is
too great for you to handle alone. If by your own power
you were able to lose weight, then you wouldn't have a
weight problem. The man with the mute son was certain that he was powerless to help his boy.

Second, believe that with God's help and through His
power you can be victorious. This choice requires us to

mature in the fruit of the Spirit of faithfulness. The man with the mute son pursued Jesus on behalf of his boy because he knew that only Christ could help him.

And finally, with sincere humility, ask the Lord to remove your doubt. Doubt can be eliminated through earnest prayer. The man with the mute son did not ignore his doubt. Instead he brought it to the Lord with honesty and openness. And just like this desperate father, when we feel doubt begin to surface, we ought to be quick to cry out, "Lord, help my unbelief."

FIRST COMES FAITH

The experiences of Moses, the apostle Thomas, John the Baptist and the man with the mute son show us that doubt will come during times of discouragement. Faith is what distinguishes this "innocent" type of doubt from the more serious form of doubt. The latter signifies an absence of faith while the former relates to a test of faith. On one occasion when Jesus encountered some Jews in the temple, they revealed their absence of faith in Him:

> Then came the Feast of Dedication at Jerusalem. It was winter, and Jesus was in the temple area walking in Solomon's Colonnade. The Jews gathered around him, saying, "How long will you keep us in suspense? If you are the Christ, tell us plainly."
>
> —JOHN 10:22–24

In the King James Version, the Jews' question reads, "How long dost thou make us to doubt?" In this case, their doubt reflects a total absence of faith. The Jews were challenging Jesus to provide proof of who He was, not because they were feeling defeat or confusion about the Messiah's identity, as in the case of the apostle Thomas. Instead, their doubt was a manifestation of a spirit of unbelief. There was no way for them to *grow* in their faith in Jesus Christ because they had no faith in Christ to begin with. Jesus' reply to their question reveals their true nature. He tells them:

> I did tell you, but you do not believe. The miracles I do in my Father's name speak for me, but you do not believe because you are not my sheep. My sheep listen to my voice; I know them and they follow me.
>
> —JOHN 10:25–27

Jesus never responded to believers in the way He did to those who did not believe in Him. A *believer* who doubts does not forsake his trust in Christ—he is still a sheep in the fold. His belief in Christ provides evidence of the faith that dwells in him. The doubt, then, becomes an indication that the faith needs strengthening; it does not denote its absence. Do you recall the man with the mute son? His plea to Christ was, "I do believe [first comes faith]; help me overcome my unbelief [deal with the doubt]."

An unbeliever, on the other hand, has no faith in Christ to begin with. And like the Jews in this passage, the unbeliever's doubt is a reflection of an absence of faith. According to this passage, an unbeliever does not listen to the Lord and does not follow (or obey) the Lord. Listening and obedience, however imperfectly, give evidence of our trust in Christ.

Performing religious rituals (including the ritual of attending church) will not by themselves give you faith. The Jews in this passage were themselves "attending church"—they challenged Christ inside of the temple. They performed the rituals of religion, but they had no faith. Unfortunately, people today sometimes *think* they have faith simply because they go through the motions of religion.

But unless you have accepted Christ as your Savior, the fruit of the Spirit of faithfulness does not dwell within you, nor do any of the fruit of the Spirit of God. You can only deal with doubt by taking it to the Lord, as we discussed. This privilege of casting your burden of doubt upon the shoulders of Jesus only comes when you choose to place your faith first in Christ.

COUNTING THE COST

How much faith do you need in order to be successful in weight loss? Jesus told His disciples, "If you have faith as small as a mustard seed, you can say to this mountain, 'Move from here to there' and it will move. Nothing will be impossible for you" (Matt. 17:20). Your lack of faith may not be the problem if you are struggling with weight problems. For some people it is not a matter of weak faith or strong doubt. The real problem is a failure to consider the cost before beginning the weight loss venture.

In the fourteenth chapter of the Gospel of Luke, Jesus teaches an important consideration of becoming a disciple:

Suppose one of you wants to build a tower. Will

he not first sit down and estimate the cost to see if
he has enough money to complete it? For if he
lays the foundation and is not able to finish it,
everyone who sees it will ridicule him, saying,
"This fellow began to build and was not able to
finish." Or suppose a king is about to go to war
against another king. Will he not first sit down
and consider whether he is able with ten thousand men to oppose the one coming against him
with twenty thousand?

—LUKE 14:28–31

In this passage Jesus is making the point that following Him is not easy—it involves a great price. Before
a decision is made to become a disciple, the cost has to
be counted. As the disciple grows in understanding, he
or she becomes better equipped to handle the challenges of being a disciple. Otherwise, when trials and
challenges come, the unprepared follower will be
inclined to turn away.

At the start of the journey, the ill-prepared disciple is
confident that following Christ is something he or she
should do, but when the going gets tough, they lose
their courage to go on. Had they counted the cost from
the beginning, they would have known to expect difficulty and wouldn't have been caught off-guard when
challenges came.

Let's apply this same principle of counting the cost to
weight loss and the fruit of the Spirit of faithfulness. I
believe that in most cases of weight loss failure, the
issue is not that the faith is small, but rather that the
cost was never properly counted.

We have already discussed how food is used to meet

needs other than that of nourishing our bodies. It is used to relieve the symptoms of depression, to counter stress and for other unacceptable purposes. So before starting a weight loss program, it's crucial to first determine the role that food is playing in our lives. If food has a level of significance beyond that of nourishing the physical body, then part of counting the cost is to acknowledge this as a problem and then devise a strategy to resolve it.

If, for instance, you eat during periods of stress, then you first need to take steps to be able to manage stress effectively—*before* you begin a weight loss program. These considerations have to be done beforehand, because the things that generate stress will not change just because you have decided to eat cauliflower instead of candy bars. So part of counting the cost might include enrolling in a stress management course or, better yet, improving the quality of your prayer life.

Counting the cost might require you to evaluate your relationships and accept that some of them need to change. Many times friendships are based on things that are shared in common, even if those things are superficial. Rich people tend to have rich friends. Single people often have single friends. And overweight people, quite commonly, have overweight friends.

When the common denominator of the relationship changes, you can expect that the relationship will change as well. In other words, if the only thing that seals the friendship is that you both are overweight, then when one friend loses weight, the foundation is destroyed and the relationship will suffer. Part of counting the cost in this scenario is first to accept that the relationship might be affected. If it is worth salvaging, then make an effort to build the relationship on a different foundation. If it is not worth salvaging (and some aren't, especially if your friend wants you to remain overweight), then count the cost and accept that your friendship will likely dissolve.

Counting the cost must include a full understanding and an acceptance that the dietary and lifestyle changes will not be temporary, but permanent. This fact is probably the most difficult part of counting the cost. It is certainly the reason why so many people regain weight after successfully losing. Then they become discouraged by their failure, and the discouragement leads to doubt. They might decide not to try again, never acknowledging that the reason for their failure was that they did not count the cost of permanent change.

Coming to terms with the end of a lifestyle is difficult. The old way of eating and living is gone forever, and a new lifestyle has to be learned. While this can be a bitter pill to swallow, it is nevertheless a truth that is a necessary component of counting the cost. It has been my sad experience that it sometimes takes a health tragedy such as a heart attack to make a person finally understand that the lifestyle changes must be permanent.

The Bible says, "Faith by itself, if it is not accompanied by action, is dead" (James 2:17). The fruit of the Spirit of faithfulness must be accompanied by the action of counting the cost. Failure to count the cost and to work actively at overcoming those things that have kept you overweight inevitably lead to weight regain and weight cycling. This pattern leads to discouragement and doubt.

I encourage you to consider what weight loss is going

to cost you. Are you prepared to pay the price? Faith alone is not enough without considering the cost. Once that decision is made, you can expect your faithful Savior to help you make the changes necessary for permanent weight loss to be your testimony. He is able and willing to help you overcome all the obstacles that seem like mountains in your life keeping you from your weight loss goals. His gentle persuasion will enable you to live in victory for the rest of your life.

Eight

The Fruit of the Spirit Is *Gentleness . . .*

Through patience a ruler can be persuaded, and a gentle tongue can break a bone.

—PROVERBS 25:15

One of my best friends is a dermatologist whom I met in medical school. I recall one of the stories she told me about a teenage patient of hers who had a bad case of acne. She placed this young lady on a specific treatment regimen and scheduled a follow-up appointment a few weeks later. When the girl returned to her office, her skin looked worse instead of better.

My friend asked her troubled young patient what happened, questioning her to find out if she had adhered to the instructions. The girl initially insisted that she had followed every directive, but later admitted that she chose to ignore one small recommendation. Instead of using cool water to rinse her face, she was using very hot water. She mistakenly assumed that hot water would provide her with a better cleansing and improve her skin. But the hot water did more to irritate her skin than clean it. My friend gave her young patient a kindhearted rebuke. The girl learned through experience that some things respond better to gentle treatment.

In this chapter, I want to focus on some of the

"ungentle" things we do to our bodies in an effort to lose weight. Most of these methods are not recommended (some are even dangerous); others are acceptable therapy provided there is professional supervision. In the end, I hope to convince you that the best approach to weight loss is the gentle approach. If you are consistent and patient with the gentle approach, you can expect to see results.

SETTING A GOAL

The first step in the "gentle" approach to weight loss is to set some reasonable goals and objectives. I often tell my church-based weight loss group (The Ex-Gravediggers) that no one should strive to look like a Barbie doll. Vanity is not allowed in our sessions. Our objectives are twofold: to improve the health of those participants who already have weight-related illnesses, and to maintain the health (through disease prevention) of those participants who don't have weight-related illnesses.

These objectives can be reached *without* reaching the "ideal body weight" found on life insurance tables. The concept of an ideal body weight began in the 1920s, when tables were created that indicated the average weight for height that was considered ideal in terms of mortality. In the late 1950s, the Build and Blood Pressure Study combined height and weight data from enrollees in twenty-six life insurance companies. The 1959 Metropolitan Life Insurance Company Desirable Body Weight Table was derived with information obtained in this study. Naturally, a life insurance company would identify an "ideal" weight as the weight associated with the lowest mortality. This made good business sense.

But research has shown that there are health benefits associated with even modest degrees of weight loss. The 1995 Dietary Guidelines for Americans states that, "Weight losses of only 5–10 percent of body weight may improve many of the problems associated with overweight, such as high blood pressure and type 2 diabetes. Even a smaller loss can make a difference."[1]

In tangible terms, if you are a female between the ages of twenty-five and fifty-nine, 5 feet 4 inches tall, and start out weighing 200 pounds, a loss of 5 to 10 percent will bring you down to somewhere between 180 and 190 pounds. This still places you in the category of obese, and it is far from the goal weights listed on the 1983 Metropolitan Height-Weight Table, which are 114–127 pounds for a small frame, 124–138 pounds for a medium frame and 134–151 pounds for a large frame—*fully dressed*. But there are clear health benefits to losing those ten to twenty pounds. And we cannot ignore these benefits.

Similarly, our approach to obesity has changed in that there is more emphasis placed on the importance of *maintaining* long-term weight loss and *preventing* long-term weight gain. The Institute of Medicine of the National Academy of Science suggests that we rethink our concept of success: "Successful long-term weight control by our definition means losing at least 5 percent of body weight...and keeping it below our definition of successful weight loss for at least one year."[2]

Since health benefits are achieved with even modest degrees of weight loss, I recommend an initial goal of a

10 percent reduction at a rate of a pound or two per week through diet and exercise. Once this goal is reached, I advise patients to maintain their loss for several months to a year before attempting to lose any more. That is a gentle approach to weight loss that is reasonable and can bring good permanent results. There are hazards to less gentle approaches to weight loss.

BINGEING AND PURGING

Emaciated young girls who think they are fat are not the only ones who suffer with eating disorders. By definition, anyone diagnosed with anorexia nervosa is thin. But this is not so with bulimia nervosa. Bulimics can be thin, normal weight or even overweight. The *Diagnostic and Statistical Manual of Mental Disorders*, fourth edition, sets guidelines for making all psychiatric diagnoses. It lists the criteria in the following chart as necessary for making the diagnosis of bulimia nervosa.[3]

BULIMIA CHARACTERISTICS

1. Recurrent episodes of binge eating. An episode of binge eating is characterized by both of the following:

    ℘ Eating, in a discrete period of time (e.g., within any two-hour period), an amount of food that is definitely larger than most people would eat during a similar period of time and under similar circumstances.

ℂ A sense of lack of control over
eating during the episode (e.g., a
feeling that one cannot stop eating
or control what or how much one
is eating).

2. Recurrent inappropriate compensatory behavior
to prevent weight gain, such as self-induced vomiting, misuse of laxatives, diuretics (water pills) or
other medications; fasting; or excessive exercise.

3. The binge eating and inappropriate compensatory behaviors both occur on average at least
twice a week for three months.

4. Self-evaluation is unduly influenced by body
shape and weight.

5. The disturbance does not occur exclusively
during episodes of anorexia nervosa.

Specific types:

ℂ **Purging type:** The person regularly
engages in self-induced vomiting or
the misuse of laxatives or diuretics.

ℂ **Non-purging type:** The person uses
other inappropriate compensatory
behaviors, such as fasting or excessive exercise, but does not regularly
engage in self-induced vomiting or
the misuse of laxatives or diuretics.

~~~

Since bulimics tend to binge and purge in secret, and
since their body weight does not draw much attention

(unlike the anorexic), they are often successful at hiding their problem from others. There is a high rate of alcohol and drug abuse among bulimics, and depression tends to be quite severe, making suicide a definite risk. Conventional treatment is often unsuccessful, with as many as 40 percent of treated patients still engaging in bulimic behavior after eighteen months of therapy. For overweight bulimics, addressing the eating disorder takes precedence over weight loss. But all too commonly the healthcare provider who is consulted for weight loss—be it a physician, nurse or dietician—is unaware of the eating disorder, and the bingeing and purging continue.

FAD DIETS

One of the reasons why the weight loss industry is so lucrative is because we are willing to spend money on fad diets that promise short-term results and not as willing to make a lifelong commitment to healthy eating and regular exercise. There is a quality in human nature that desires "something for nothing." It's this tendency that makes fad diets so appealing—they promise a quick and easy solution to a complex and difficult problem.

There are literally hundreds of fad diets available. Some are based on a single food item where the dieter is allowed to eat the particular food in excess but limits everything else. Other fad diets are based on a specific nutrient like protein. Still others have no rhyme or reason and are based on things that aren't related to food at all. The following are examples of just a few of the more popular fad diets. They cannot be classified as gentle approaches to weight loss.

The grapefruit diet

The specific instructions for this diet vary depending on the source, but in general, the plan requires that a whole or half of a grapefruit be eaten before each meal. The dieter is also encouraged to drink lots of coffee or tea. This diet is based on the premise that grapefruit contains an enzyme that burns fat. In reality, no such enzyme has ever been discovered. Grapefruit is a good source of vitamin C and folic acid and should be part of any healthy diet, but like any other food, it shouldn't be eaten exclusively or in excess. If you happen to lose weight on this diet, then it is because grapefruit is a low-calorie, low-fat food—not because of any mystery enzyme.

Everyone who drinks coffee will attest that caffeine has a diuretic effect—it causes excessive urination. So "success" with the grapefruit diet may simply result from loss of water weight, which will re-accumulate once you replenish your body's fluids.

The cabbage soup diet

This diet appeals to people who want to lose weight fast. It claims that up to ten pounds can be shed in a one-week period of time, without ever feeling hungry. That claim alone should generate suspicion, but those who want a "quick-fix" often lose sight of what makes (or doesn't make) common sense. This is also a single-food diet. Instead of grapefruit, the dieter is allowed to eat unlimited quantities of cabbage soup. The plan also recommends caffeine-containing beverages so, once again, any drop in the scale is likely to represent water weight.

High-protein diets

These diets are based on the premise that carbohydrates make us hungry, and this leads to overeating. The proposed solution is to eliminate carbohydrates from the diet and substitute them with large quantities of protein and fat. This is in direct opposition to the recommendations of the American Dietetic Association—remember that carbohydrates form the foundation of the food pyramid.

One obvious problem with this diet is that it will lack many of the vitamins and nutrients that are found in carbohydrate foods. A more serious consequence is that when carbohydrates are eliminated, the body generates excessive amounts of ketones, the chemical by-product of fat metabolism. High levels of ketones can cause headaches, nausea, fatigue and dizziness. Since ketones are generated during times of starvation, they act as signals that instruct the body to slow down its rate of metabolism and preserve energy. Consequently, once you stop the diet, you tend to regain quickly any weight that was lost because of this reduction in your metabolic rate.

Fad diets unrelated to food

Blood type. In recent years I have had at least a dozen patients ask me (somewhat surreptitiously) if I would check their blood type. This is not considered a "routine" laboratory test, and I wondered why there was such a new surge of interest. I later learned that one popular diet recommends that certain foods be eaten (or avoided) based on the person's blood type. The theory is that the different blood types evolved over time, so those individuals with more primitive blood types are better equipped to handle primitive foods like meat. Individuals with blood types that evolved more recently are better equipped to handle sophisticated foods like vegetables.

The flaw in this theory is that those components in our food that supposedly react to our blood are either destroyed through the process of cooking, or they are destroyed by the digestive enzymes in our gastrointestinal track. As a result, these food components never even enter the bloodstream to interact with our particular blood type.

Deep breathing. There's another weight loss plan that recommends deep breathing exercises. This weight loss plan claims that the extra oxygen taken into your body will generate more energy for fat metabolism. However, this theory does not line up with basic physiology. In simple terms, whether you sigh, pant or yawn, a calorie is still a calorie, and the extra calories are stored as fat. Oxygen will not eliminate the need to eat less food.

Hormonal imbalance. Another popular diet postulates that obesity is the end result of a hormonal imbalance. It claims that eating certain foods will somehow correct this imbalance and facilitate weight loss. Would that the epidemic of obesity resulted from a few wayward glands secreting improper amounts of hormones. Unfortunately, the problem is not one of hormones; it's one of calories.

VERY-LOW-CALORIE DIETS
AND STARVATION DIETS

There is a potential (but major) problem that arises when we set out to reduce the number of calories consumed each day, and that is whether or not the recommended daily allowance of vitamins and minerals will be reached. Diets consisting of as little as 1200 calories per day can be nutritionally complete, provided those calories are not wasted on foods with minimal or no nutritional value. A diet comprised of less than 1200 calories per day runs the risk of being nutritionally inadequate and should be undertaken only with a physician's supervision.

Starvation diets consist of zero calories—no fat, no protein and no carbohydrates. Those unfortunates who are placed on these diets are given enough water to avoid dehydration, and they receive supplements of vitamins, minerals and electrolytes (chemicals such as potassium, calcium, sodium and magnesium that are essential for normal cellular function). Cardiovascular complications are the major concern with starvation diets. Along with abnormalities in the electrocardiogram, there are many case reports of patients on starvation diets dying suddenly from various disturbances in the heart's conduction and rhythm.

Very-low-calorie diets are usually liquid meals, often in the form of "shakes," that replace a regular, solid food meal. Protein-sparing modified fasts are very-low-calorie diets that *do* contain solid foods, but in the form of high-protein, low-fat, low-carbohydrate meals. Very-low-calorie diets typically provide 400–800 calories per day, along with a supplement of vitamins, minerals, electrolytes and all of the essential fatty acids and amino acids. These diets should be undertaken only with a healthcare provider's supervision and should be used *only* in the case of obesity—they are not recommended for cosmetic weight reduction. In addition, it is recommended that six months of behavior modification (including exercise instruction) and nutrition education be a part of the overall plan in order to reduce the risk of weight regain.

Very-low-calorie diets are safer than starvation diets, though there have been case reports of patients experiencing abnormal cardiac rhythms, and even cardiac arrest, while on these diets.

Outside of the obvious health risks, fad diets, starvation diets and very-low-calorie diets are impractical since they cannot be followed for an indefinite amount of time. More importantly, they fail to address the underlying psychological, emotional and spiritual issues that lead to obesity.

WEIGHT LOSS MEDICATIONS

Weight loss medications have been around for years. Older drugs worked by suppressing the appetite or by speeding up the metabolism. Amphetamine was the prototype weight loss medication of the 1950s and 1960s. Use was limited by adverse side effects, along with a significant risk of addiction. This potential for addiction served to stigmatize the pharmacological approach to weight loss for many years. But in the past decade or so, much research has been devoted to the development of new drugs. Some of these drugs have been approved for long-term use; others have been withdrawn from the market because of safety concerns.

In 1992, reports of successful weight loss through use of a combination of two drugs, fenfluramine and phentermine, gained widespread attention. The "fen-phen" combination took the country by storm. The demand for these drugs was so great that weight loss "clinics" began popping up all over the place. For a sizable fee, you could leave one of these establishments with a coveted fen-phen prescription, regardless of whether you needed it or not. Many "patients" who were prescribed fen-phen were *not* obese; some weren't even overweight. It was widely prescribed for cosmetic purposes in the absence of solid medical indications.

In 1996, the drug dexfenfluramine received approval for use as a weight loss medication. Until this time, the Food and Drug Administration had not approved any medications for weight loss for twenty-three years. Unlike fenfluramine, dexfenfluramine was authorized for continuous use up to a year. The drug was so popular that 3.3 million prescriptions were written from June 1996 to April 1997. In the spring of 1997, reports began to surface that people using fenfluramine and dexfenfluramine were developing abnormalities in their heart valves. Soon thereafter, the FDA withdrew both drugs from the market.[4]

There are currently eight drugs that have FDA approval for weight loss. Two of these, sibutramine and orlistat, were released subsequent to the withdrawal of fenfluramine and dexfenfluramine; they are the only ones with FDA approval for long-term use. The others are approved for short-term intervals of three months or less.

Sibutramine works as an appetite suppressant. It, like some antidepressant drugs, alters the balance of chemicals in the brain such as norepinephrine, serotonin and dopamine. Studies have shown that patients taking sibutramine were able to lose 7 to 8 percent of their initial body weight over the course of a year, compared to a 1 to 2 percent loss in patients taking a placebo.[5]

Some of the side effects of sibutramine include headache, dry mouth, constipation and insomnia. There have been reports of elevations in blood pressure and pulse rate; for this reason people using sibutramine should have these monitored at regular intervals.

Orlistat works in an entirely different manner. It has no central nervous system effects and does not suppress the appetite; it works at the level of the intestine. It prevents fat from being digested in the intestine and absorbed into the bloodstream, which means that a large portion of the fat consumed is eliminated in the stool. Quite predictably, the major side effects are related to the gastrointestinal tract— oily stool, excessive gas and an inability to control bowel movements. There is also a concern that orlistat may impair the absorption of the four vitamins that require an oil-based medium to dissolve—vitamins A, D, E and K. Because of this, patients are advised to take a multivitamin supplement containing these four vitamins. Patients who respond to orlistat can expect to lose 8 to 10 percent of their initial body weight in six to twelve months.[6]

Neither sibutramine nor orlistat is approved for cosmetic weight reduction. These drugs should only be prescribed to patients who are obese or to patients who are overweight and have weight-related medical conditions.

THE SURGICAL APPROACH

Because of the high rate of failure with diet plans (even plans that are safe and medically supervised) and the limited efficacy with even long-term use of weight loss medications (at best, a 10 percent reduction of the initial body weight), the surgical approach to weight loss is rapidly becoming more popular and acceptable. As a point of clarification, liposuction is cosmetic surgery—not weight loss surgery. It is a procedure that is done for the sole purpose of changing the contour of the body. It does not remove large amounts of fat, or fat from inside the abdominal cavity. The ideal candidate for liposuction is a healthy adult with a localized area of fat underneath the skin.

Liposuction is the most commonly performed cosmetic procedure in the United States. Nearly 150,000 people had it done in 1997—a threefold increase from the numbers reported in 1992.[7] The thighs and hips are the most popular spots, but it can be done almost anywhere on the body including the abdomen, legs, knees, ankles, buttocks, face, neck, arms and breasts. Liposuction is purportedly safe, but since it is not mandatory that physicians report complications related to the procedure, the incidence of adverse outcomes (including death) is unknown.[8]

In very general terms, weight loss surgery works to either decrease the capacity of the stomach, limit the absorption of food or both. Patients considered for weight loss surgery should meet several criteria. In addition to extreme obesity (or lesser degrees of obesity if weight-related medical conditions are present), patients should have tried and failed at several traditional weight loss methods. They should be carefully screened for any psychiatric disturbances such as an eating disorder, and they should fully understand that surgery does not eliminate the need for lifestyle changes—diet and exercise are still required to insure long-term success.

Gastric bypass surgery is a safe procedure with impressive long-term results. This procedure, like many other operations, can now be done laparoscopically. The laparoscopic approach has been gaining in popularity because of the smaller incision, fewer complications, less pain and a shorter hospital stay. The average gastric bypass patient loses two-thirds of excess body weight (or one-third of total weight) within one year. Most patients maintain a 60 percent loss of excess body weight at five years and 50 percent at ten years following their operations.

Complications of this surgery include those that are directly related to the procedure such as the risks of surgery, general anesthesia and problems related to the incision site (wound infections, improper healing and hernias), as well as long-term adverse effects like vitamin deficiencies, protein malnutrition and osteoporosis. With a balanced diet and regular follow-up, these long-term complications can be avoided.

My personal philosophy

I am often asked my opinion regarding weight loss medications and weight loss surgery. People who know that I am a Christian and know that I believe in the power of the Holy Spirit are curious to know whether I prescribe sibutramine and orlistat, and whether I refer patients to surgeons. The idea of taking a pill or having a major operation to lose weight seems to run counter to all the spiritual principles that I emphasize, especially the principle of self-control. The answer to both questions is yes—I *do* write prescriptions, and I *do* send patients for surgical evaluations, even Christian patients. Am I, then, a hypocrite? Is it possible to strike a balance between my faith and my practice?

I take the following stance when it comes to medications and operations. I firmly believe that it is possible to lose weight through implementing lifestyle changes such as following a healthy diet and getting adequate exercise. I believe that the power necessary to implement these changes is available to the Christian through the indwelling Holy Spirit. But I cannot ignore reality. And the reality is that the principles that I have outlined in this book require a level of spiritual maturity that cannot be attained overnight. Many of my patients, and some of the women in my weight loss group, are "babes in Christ." They are actively working to grow in their faith, but growth takes time—sometimes years, decades or even a lifetime.

So I am faced with a dilemma: Do I do nothing other than wait for them to grow strong enough in their faith so that they can lose weight through the power of the Holy Spirit alone? Or do I provide them with assistance in the form of medications and operations *while* they mature in their faith? I have selected the second option for one reason—the consequences of weight-related diseases don't wait for spiritual growth. I would do my patients a disservice if I refused to provide them with therapy and waited for them to mature spiritually while diseases such as type 2 diabetes, hypertension, arthritis and sleep apnea wreaked havoc on their bodies.

I believe in the power of the Holy Spirit, and I strongly recommend the gentle approach to weight loss through diet and exercise alone. But I must also use wisdom and consider each patient's circumstances. I would encourage you to seek God in prayer if you are contemplating weight loss medications or if you are seriously considering surgery. Neither decision should be made lightly, but only after you've sought godly counsel and found peace through prayer.

Nine

The Fruit of
the Spirit Is
Self-Control . . .

*Like a city whose walls are broken
down is a man who lacks self-control.*
—PROVERBS 25:28

This scripture compares a lack of self-control to a city whose walls are broken down. Because our modern cities do not have walls, this proverb may be difficult for us to understand. We need to ask the question "What is the significance of a city with broken-down walls?" in order to grasp the comparison to our lack of self-control.

Like David and Goliath and Jonah and the fish, the Old Testament account of Joshua and the battle of Jericho is very familiar to most of us. As children we sang songs about how Joshua "fit" the battle of Jericho and "the walls came tumblin' down." Even beyond Sunday school classes and Junior Church, the account of this famous battle is a commonly used sermon topic because it is so rich in biblical principles.

The Bible describes Jericho as a walled city that was "tightly shut up because of the Israelites. No one went out and no one came in" (Josh. 6:1). In our era of sophisticated warfare that utilizes computerized surveillance systems and "smart" bombs, the idea that a stone wall might afford much protection to a city's inhabitants, or that it would represent a formidable obstacle to those who wanted to do battle with them, is hard to fathom. But that was indeed the case with Jericho.

The principal cities of biblical times were surrounded by walls that were 15 to 25 feet thick and 25 feet high, often with observation towers built at each corner. Some walls had trenches in the front to provide additional protection. A city with a strong wall was virtually impregnable to attack, and the inhabitants lived in peace. If the walls of a city were compromised, the city became open to enemy attack. The land itself and everything inside the city—the money, the livestock and the people—were vulnerable without the protection of the city wall.

The significance of the walled city becomes clear in the proverb as we understand that a lack of self-control will bring destruction to our lives just as broken walls brought destruction to a city. The fruit of the Spirit of self-control protects us as the city wall protected the city. Without it, we become vulnerable to our enemy, Satan, whose purpose is to steal, kill and destroy (John 10:10).

> *A lack of self-control will bring destruction to our lives.*

It is true that the walls confined the citizens and restricted their freedom, just as self-control requires that we place restraints and limitations upon ourselves. But for the inhabitants of walled cities, the benefits of protection greatly exceeded the inconvenience of being confined. This is also true regarding the fruit of self-control. The restraints it requires bring great benefits of protection from self-destructive lifestyles.

Too often we have a tendency to focus on all the things we're *missing* when we practice self-control, rather than all the benefits of being *protected* from things that will harm us. This tendency to dwell on the limitations and restrictions associated with self-control is part of human nature—we're prone to focus on the negative in every circumstance that requires us to practice restraint.

For example, God has placed the biblical requirement to practice self-control over our sexual drives. His intent is to protect us from the inevitable destruction of our lives without this restraint. People who engage in premarital sex will justify fornication based on what they're missing, failing to recognize the many benefits that come with abstinence apart from marriage, including protection from sexually transmitted diseases, unwanted pregnancy and a disrupted fellowship with God because of sin.

Once our protective wall of self-control is compromised in any area, we begin a vicious cycle that leads to greater and greater damage to our already crumbling wall. The smallest crack in our wall allows Satan to enter and tempt us. Caught off-guard (from a lack of self-control), we are vulnerable to temptation that is far more intense than if our wall was intact.

Once we yield to a lack of restraint in any area, the wall of self-control crumbles even more, opening us up to even greater temptation. The end result is a complete lack of self-control. In the case of obesity, losing control might sound like, "Well, as heavy as I am, what difference will one more scoop of ice cream make?" And the walls come tumbling down.

As with all the fruit of the Spirit, the secret to victory is learning to yield to the Holy Spirit's power within us. Only the Lord can restore a wall that's been destroyed. We must never believe that self-control is accomplished through our own will power and determination. As we have discussed, we must learn to rely totally upon the supernatural power that comes from the fruit of the Spirit, choosing to live in dependency on Him.

ACCOUNTABILITY AND RESPONSIBILITY

Self-control is the only fruit of the Spirit with a bad reputation. No matter what your theology, the other eight fruit sound pretty good. Even an atheist or agnostic would probably agree that love, joy, peace, patience, kindness, goodness, faithfulness and gentleness are character traits that are worth striving for. But when it comes to self-control we perceive the aspect of restraint that sounds negative.

"If it feels good, do it."

We are inclined to ignore it, scoff at it or be rather neutral about it. We view self-control as a nice, but unobtainable ideal that we may speak of in theory but are incapable of practicing. These are usual responses from non-Christians and Christians alike. The end result of this reasoning is that, instead of practicing self-control, we succumb to the doctrine of indulgence that says, "If it feels good, do it."

So rather than take charge of our impulses and

subdue them, we look for "safe" ways to indulge them. "Think *before* you drink" is the catch phrase for a popular alcoholic beverage company. But they aren't suggesting that you seriously consider the option of not drinking at all. And the slogan wasn't created to encourage you to drink in moderation, making a decision beforehand to keep things under control. Rather, the slogan serves to remind you to have a designated driver to get you home in your drunken stupor. The unwritten message is that it is acceptable to lose control, yielding to the lusts of the flesh. What is not acceptable are the *consequences* of yielding—a DUI citation or a potentially fatal car accident.

We have totally rejected the notion of self-control when it comes to sexuality. Rather than exercise restraint, we encourage everyone—even children—to practice "safe" sex. The message we are sending to our youth is that the self-control abstinence requires is not a virtue, but an archaic ideal that has no place in the twenty-first century. We've shown them through example that sexual impulses ought not to be controlled, but simply indulged in a "safe" manner. And the best way to insure that everyone is "safe" is to teach our children the proper way to use a condom; that way, when you "give in" or "yield," you'll avoid getting pregnant or catching an incurable disease (which is a false assumption, because condoms do not always protect against sexually transmitted diseases).

It's time for us to reevaluate our attitude toward self-control. When I started this book, I remember telling my husband how relieved I was that the fruit of the Spirit of self-control came last. Perhaps by then I could muster the courage to say those things that are unpopular but convicting.

Self-control is one of the most profound secrets to walking in liberty from bondages of all kinds, especially the bondages of being overweight and of obesity. The first step in maturing in the fruit of self-control is to accept responsibility and become accountable for your choices and actions. Simply put, it will be impossible for you to take control of a situation (i.e., your weight) if you believe the situation is totally beyond your control.

Arguing against the evidence

The statement I am most likely to hear from my overweight and obese patients is that they don't eat very much. Even if this statement is true in the present, it was not always the case. If you are overweight or obese, at *some* point during your lifetime you consumed more calories than you needed. On what evidence do I base this fact? The numbers on the scale.

> *Self-control is one of the most profound secrets to walking in liberty.*

Arguing against the evidence does nothing to solve the problem. If, for example, I noticed that most of the plants in my garden were turning dry and brown, I might call an expert to get some advice. The master gardener would more than likely say that I need to give my plants more water. Now I could argue with him and claim that I give the plants plenty of water. I could show him my watering schedule, show him the design of my sprinkling system and complain that he had obviously made the wrong assessment.

But the expert is only going by the evidence: dry, brown plants. My defense of my watering practices does nothing to change the evidence. I would be better served (and my plants would be better served) if I became less defensive and accepted responsibility for the state of my garden. Maybe I'm *not* giving an adequate amount, or maybe I'm watering at the wrong time of day and much of the water is evaporating, or maybe I need to amend my soil so that it will absorb the water more effectively. Not until I accept responsibility and become accountable to the expert can I solve the problem.

One of the reasons people struggle to lose weight and avoid taking responsibility for being overweight is that they became overweight during childhood (or even during the infant or toddler years). They *didn't* have full control of their eating, and they *aren't* responsible for the poor eating habits established by their parents or caretakers. Now their bodies have an established "set point," that is, they are extremely efficient at conserving calories and it becomes very difficult, seemingly impossible, to lose weight.

In this case, it is important to acknowledge the actions of others and accept that their decisions contributed to your problem. In order for you to reverse the results of their actions in your past, however, you will have to assume responsibility for your present and future. You are now responsible for *un*doing (to the best of your ability) the mistakes your parents made. It will be *your* responsibility to engage in regular exercise to improve your metabolism and break those weight plateaus, and *you* will be responsible for changing those unhealthy eating habits that were established during your childhood.

Whatever the root of the problem that has caused your obesity or being overweight, your role now is to become accountable and accept responsibility to develop the fruit of self-control. As you allow the Holy Spirit to work in your life, you will find the strength to make right choices and become responsible for your actions.

> *Arguing against the evidence does nothing to solve the problem.*

My experience has taught me that for most overweight people there is more involved in their problem than a mother who gave too much candy when they were little. The problem may lie in the quantity of the food (large serving sizes), the quality of the food (high fat content, "empty" calories) or both, with the end result that more calories are consumed than are required.

Food requirements are relative to personal metabolism needs. What may be an appropriate amount of food for a lean adolescent boy who plays basketball several hours a day and is in the middle of a growth spurt is entirely *inappropriate* for a middle-aged woman who sits at a desk all day and does not exercise. It is imperative that people understand their body's needs for nourishment and exercise self-control in meeting those needs. It is also important to understand that those needs change during different stages of our lives.

I am not an advocate of severely structured diet plans, the types that tell you exactly what to eat for every meal, each day of the week. I think that eating should involve some degree of spontaneity and flexibility. But I do find structured diet plans particularly helpful when I encounter patients who insist that they don't eat much food. Using a sample diet can help to bring objectivity to their evaluation of how much food they eat.

This is a recommended breakfast, lunch, dinner and snack from a typical low-calorie diet plan. Pay particular attention to the serving sizes and the relative absence of foods that are comprised of empty calories (those foods and condiments that are high in calories but have no real nutritional value). This is a typical day's menu from a 1600-calorie plan:

TYPICAL DAILY MENU

BREAKFAST
1 cup oatmeal
½ cup fruit cocktail
1 cup plain, low-fat yogurt
Black coffee or tea with lemon

LUNCH
2 slices whole-wheat bread
2 oz. turkey-ham and 1 oz. low-fat cheese
⅛ avocado sliced
alfalfa sprouts
1 tsp. mayonnaise
½ cup baby carrots

2 tablespoons nonfat dressing for dipping
   carrots
1 apple
Water or non-caloric beverage

DINNER

5 oz. chicken leg, no skin, baked
1 cup whole-wheat pasta
4 Tbsp. low-fat vinaigrette (2 Tbsp. for mari-
   nade for chicken and 2 Tbsp. to toss with
   pasta)
1 cup broccoli and 1 cup zucchini, steamed
   and tossed with pasta
8 oz. 1 percent milk

SNACK

1 cup cantaloupe
¼ cup 1 percent cottage cheese

~~~~~

Most patients who review this typical 1600-calorie menu are amazed at the difference between the amount of food they *should* be eating and what they actually eat. In many cases, empty calories are a major problem. Snack foods, chips, sweets (e.g., candy, cake, doughnuts, ice cream) and sodas are not only the sources of empty calories, but they tend to be the forgotten foods—foods we eat without paying much attention to the fact that we are eating them.

When it comes to easily eliminated calories, sodas top the list. A can of soda contains an average of one hundred fifty calories. The math is simple: If you drink two 12-ounce cans of soda each day, you have consumed

three hundred empty calories. If you are following a
1500-calorie diet, that means that 20 percent of your
allowed calories have been wasted on soda. If you drink
three 12-ounce cans, you have consumed 30 percent of
your allowed calories in soda pop. Keep in mind that
many fast-food restaurants offer large drinks that contain
42 ounces of soda pop—their "super" sizes. By our calcu-
lations, that one drink would have approximately 525
empty calories, or 35 percent of what's allowed in a
1500-calorie diet.

*It is imperative
that people
understand their body's
needs for nourishment
and exercise self-control
in meeting those needs.*

In order to live a life governed by self-control, we
must be willing to be accountable for our choices and
accept responsibility for our actions. I remember taking
care of an obese patient who had type 2 diabetes that
was pretty difficult to control. Every visit, after being
weighed by the nurse, she'd shrug her shoulders and
shake her head in frustration. Her weight was predictably a pound or two more than it was on our
previous visit, but she was adamant in her stance that it
wasn't her fault. There was something unique about her
body that made it gain weight autonomously, independent of her desires and totally against her will.

One day while I was rushing to get to the clinic, I
passed by the hospital's gift shop at the same time that
she was exiting, and we nearly collided with one

another. Her mouth was so completely stuffed with chocolate candy that I could hardly understand her when she greeted me. She didn't even wait until she was out of the store to begin eating. I smiled and returned her greeting, but we gave one another a look that confirmed her secret: The mystery weight gain was really no mystery at all.

The prophet Hosea gave the warning, "My people are destroyed from lack of knowledge" (Hos. 4:6). Though we have the knowledge about how to improve our health, we will still be destroyed if we fail to act on the knowledge we have. We are suffering this condition because we have avoided the crucial step of accepting responsibility and accountability. When we begin taking steps toward becoming responsible and accountable for our choices and actions, we will be released from being *victims* of our circumstances to being *victorious* in our health.

VICTIM OR VICTOR

There is abundant evidence that genetics plays a role in body weight and the tendency toward obesity can be inherited. Adoption studies have shown that children whose biological parents were overweight have a higher than average likelihood of becoming overweight themselves, no matter what their adoptive parents weigh. So even if you have started eating a healthier diet and exercising regularly, if Grandpa, Grandma, Mom, Dad and all your brothers and sisters are obese, you undoubtedly have a strong genetic component that is going to work against you.

But while this is a reality, it is reassuring to know that DNA is not able to nullify the first law of thermodynamics. For those who never took physics (and for all those who took it but forgot the principles after the final exam), let me restate it:

> For any process, the difference between the heat supplied to the system and the work done by the system equals the change in the internal energy.

For our purposes, this law applies to the fact that all the calories we consume in the form of food are either burned or stored. This basic law guarantees that if we eat and absorb into our systems more calories than we utilize, those extra calories will not just disappear; they will be stored in the form of fat. We utilize calories through our bodies' normal functions—functions like a beating heart, a thinking brain and a churning stomach—and through the voluntary and involuntary use of our muscles. Of course, when engaging in regular exercise we will burn up more calories. But even when we aren't active, our muscles require a certain amount of energy to maintain posture and tone.

The obvious conclusion to this law as related to weight gain is that if we consistently consume more calories than we burn, the extra calories will be stored, and we will gain weight. If, however, we consistently eat *fewer* calories than what our bodies require, the additional calories that are needed will (ideally) come from that unused energy previously stored in the form of fat. I qualify this last statement with "ideally" because when we approach weight loss in the wrong manner, it is possible for those additional calories to come from our lean muscle tissue and not our fat stores.

Genetics plays a role in determining our body's frame—Asians tend to be smaller than Europeans, who tend to be smaller than Africans. Our genes also determine how our fat will be distributed, whether we will be "apples" with most of our weight above the waist, or "pears" with our fat stored primarily in the hips and thighs. And our genes work in establishing our bodies' "set point," that weight where we tend to plateau, beyond which it becomes difficult to lose, no matter how hard we try.

Our genes do not nullify, however, the first law of thermodynamics. For example, suppose an obese person became stranded on a deserted island where the only foods available to eat were low in fat but rich in nutrients. And suppose this food was not readily available, but was obtained only through working hard for several hours each day. And then suppose that, despite our island dweller's best efforts, there was a limit to the quantity of food available to him each day—no more than about eighteen hundred calories on a daily basis. In this hypothetical situation, even if every member of our castaway's family were obese, he would eventually lose weight.

A comfortable victim

Genetics cannot override the first law of thermodynamics. This is evident in the rapidly increasing prevalence of obesity in recent years—our genes have not changed significantly in the past few decades, but the incidence of obesity has skyrocketed. We are victims of obesity because of our lifestyles, though we try to point our fingers at an external cause for our problems. Our mentality is so victim oriented that we try to blame anything we can, irresponsibly, for circumstances that are either completely or partially under our control.

We have become so comfortable with being victims that the idea of victorious living is foreign to many Christians. Sure, we sing songs that speak of our victory in Christ, but when it comes to actually experiencing this victory in our everyday lives, we're falling short. This is because living victoriously requires a measure of self-control.

We won't know the victory in forgiving those who have hurt us until we take responsibility for our emotional responses. We won't know the victory of sexual purity until we learn to control our carnal nature. And we won't live victoriously in the area of our health until we choose to take control of our lifestyles—control over what we eat, how much we eat and how we exercise.

Are you a victim or a victor? Let the evidence speak for itself. The question to ask yourself is this: "Am I powerless in this situation?" Your answer is what determines whether your mind-set is that of a victim or a victor. If you believe that you are completely powerless, then the first step for you to take is to overcome the victim's mentality.

The person with a victim mentality resigns himself to the thought that his condition and circumstances are beyond his control. He does not believe that he has the power to alter his situation, so he will accept whatever comes his way and not make much of an effort to change things. I don't want to be misunderstood—I am not implying that bad things only happen to people with a victim mentality. Obviously that is not the case. Bad things will happen to all types of people, and many times we are confronted with circumstances that are well beyond our control. But the victim has a fatalistic attitude about everything, and he will not try to change even those things that are within his control.

A *challenging victor*

The difference between the victim and the victor lies in the way they approach circumstances, those that are changeable and those that are unchangeable. The victim will make no effort to change a potentially alterable set of circumstances, while the victor will challenge his or her situation. And when the circumstances are *unchangeable*, the victim will wallow in self-pity while the victor will rise above the circumstances.

There is an interesting dynamic in our society when it comes to the problem of obesity. On the one hand, there is the unavoidable message that we must be victorious and take control of our lifestyles. We are bombarded with ads for home exercise equipment and special offers to join the neighborhood health club. There are literally hundreds of cookbooks and culinary magazines that offer nothing but low-fat, low-calorie recipes. Many foods now come in both their original forms, as well as a "low-fat" version. And we constantly hear advice on how to live healthier lives on the radio, on television and even piped into our supermarket's sound system.

Despite this onslaught of health-related information, the incidence and prevalence of obesity continue to rise. So while we are bombarded with messages that suggest to us that we are fully capable of taking control of our lives, the actual statistics show that we're doing anything *but* taking control. The victor's mentality is promoted, but the victim's mentality prevails. The key difference between the victim and the victor is self-control.

After my second child was born, my weight came off rather steadily until I got to about ten pounds over my pre-pregnancy weight—and then it stopped. I hit a plateau. This didn't happen to me with my first child. With her, I continued to lose until all the weight was gone. So I found myself faced with a choice. I could accept the ten extra pounds as inevitable and, with the true resignation of a victim, conclude that every woman gains weight after having even one child, and I had two children.

*The key differ-
ence between the
victim and the victor is
self-control.*

But I didn't like the victim's role. And since I knew that there was no medical reason for a woman to gain weight following each pregnancy (even though we accept this as an inescapable outcome), it made my plight all the more troubling. So I evaluated my daily routine and discovered an easily correctable habit that I had picked up. During my pregnancy, I regularly stopped at the hospital gift shop at the end of the day. I would buy three "bite-sized" pieces of candy for ten cents apiece and eat them on the way to the parking lot. By the time I reached my car, I was finished with the candy.

Needless to say, after my son was born, this habit continued. It had become such a routine that I never really gave it much thought—until I hit my weight plateau. Each of those miniature pieces of candy contained seventy empty calories. So in my short walk to the parking lot, I was packing an extra two hundred ten calories, five days a week. Once I practiced a little self-control and stopped this mindless routine, I broke the plateau, the weight began to come off again, and it wasn't long before my weight was back to where I wanted it to be.

Going from victim to victor sometimes only requires that we step back, evaluate our situation and yield to the fruit of the Spirit of self-control to take the proverbial bull by the horn. Even small changes in our eating habits or our daily activity levels can make a big difference over the long run.

Our ambulatory clinic building is a state-of-the-art structure with glass-encased staircases and halls. Anyone climbing the stairs or walking the halls is clearly visible from the street, and even from various locations inside the building. I am always amazed that whenever I see the stairway, it's usually empty. It doesn't matter what time of day or what day of the week, there is usually no one climbing or descending the stairs. This amazes me because I know that I have personally advised literally hundreds of patients to increase their daily activity by using the stairs rather than the elevators. The thirty seconds it takes to climb a flight of stairs is a simple (yet, in my experience, totally disregarded) way of going from victim to victor.

The fruit of the Spirit of self-control gives us the

power to control our behavior. Because God has blessed us with this capacity, we can be sure that it is the desire of our heavenly Father that we be victors, not victims.

God gave us our human desires and appetites as a blessing; without them, we would not survive. But He does not intend for us to be governed by them. Our appetite for food sustains us, and our appetite for sex insures future generations. Our appetites are a gift from God, but we have allowed them to control us. We are like marionettes—mindless puppets having no internal power, being pulled this way and that by a string of uncontrolled desires. Instead of being in control of our desires, *our desires* control *us*.

But God, in His infinite wisdom, knew that we would have the tendency to give in to our flesh, so He gave us the fruit of the Spirit of self-control. As we draw upon the power of the Holy Spirit, we can live our lives as victors, not victims. He has given us everything we need to control our appetites. It is up to us to mature in the area of self-control and begin to enjoy this secret of living victoriously.

Handling Temptation

Temptation is the number one enemy for anyone trying to mature in the area of self-control. It is a never-ending power, an ever-present force that continuously works against us, enticing us to give up control and surrender to our impulses. Our goal in weight loss is to become *consistent resisters* of temptation. This is the only way to achieve success in the short-term and, most importantly, in the long-term. To accomplish our goals, however, we

must first understand what the Bible says about temptation and how God expects us to respond to it.

The Bible assures us that God does not entice us to
commit sinful acts: "When tempted, no one should say,
'God is tempting me.' For God cannot be tempted by
evil, nor does he tempt anyone" (James 1:13). The
Bible makes it clear that God will often test us, but He
will not entice us to commit a sin. He will allow us to
experience temptation from several sources: Satan,
people and even ourselves.

Tempted by Satan

Satan is given many names in the Bible. Along with
"enemy," "Beelzebub," "dragon" and "liar," he is also
identified as the "tempter" (c.f., Matt. 4:3; 1 Thess. 3:5).
The most familiar biblical passage where Satan acts as a
tempter is in the Book of Genesis where he convinces
Eve to eat from the tree of the Garden of Eden that was
forbidden by God.

The Gospels record the account of how Satan, as the
tempter, confronted Jesus in the wilderness to entice
Him to eat: "The devil said to him, 'If you are the Son
of God, tell this stone to become bread'" (Luke 4:3). At
this point, Jesus had been fasting for forty days and
nights. Though Jesus was divine, He was also fully
human and would have felt extreme hunger after such
a long period without food. His temptation takes on an
added significance when we realize it came at a time of
a genuine physical need.

In His response to Satan, Jesus does not deny the
truth of Satan's statement: He *was* the Son of God and
He *could* have turned the stones into bread. When
tempted, Jesus didn't tell Satan, "Oh, you're wrong; I'm

really not that hungry at all." This would have been a lie, given the circumstances. Instead He answers him with a higher truth: "It is written: 'Man does not live on bread alone'" (v. 4).

Jesus was in the wilderness, enduring hunger and denying His physical needs in order to accomplish His greater mission. When it comes to obesity and weight loss, we also have a greater mission that is more important than the mild discomfort of hunger. That mission is one of honoring our physical bodies, God's temple, by treating them in a way that promotes health, strength and longevity. Feelings of hunger should be expected with any attempt to lose weight. And when hunger hits us, we can expect Satan, the tempter, to entice us to yield. But thank God for the wonderful power of the Holy Spirit who dwells in us. When Satan comes to tempt us, we can learn the secret of yielding to the fruit of the Spirit of self-control that empowers us to resist all temptation.

The hunger issue

We have been fooled into thinking that it is possible to lose weight and keep it off without ever once experiencing hunger. Weight loss plans are promoted under the premise that you can eat what you want, never feel hungry and still shed pounds effortlessly. This is simply not true. The sooner we reject this notion, the better. Yes, there are drugs available that are designed to suppress the appetite, but these drugs should not be used indefinitely. One way or another, we have to come to terms with hunger and learn to tolerate it if we expect success.

I have a patient whose maximum weight was 230 pounds. She now weighs 170 and has maintained that weight for several years. When people ask her the secret to her success, she tells them, "Good old hunger." She experimented with a variety of different diets and weight loss plans, but they all eventually failed. Success came only when she accepted the inevitability of hunger, learned to tolerate it and took responsibility to control the impulse to eat with abandon when she felt even the mildest sensation of hunger. In addition, she paid close attention to bodily cues so that she *stopped eating* once real hunger subsided—a simple, effective approach to weight loss, grounded in the fruit of self-control.

Tempted by people

The second source of temptation is from other people, and this can be either intentional or unintentional. Some people may not know that you are trying to lose weight and will offer you things to eat in an effort to be polite. This is unintentional temptation and should be addressed by simply telling the person that you are trying to control your eating habits. A person whose motives are pure will understand and stop offering you food.

The bigger problem comes in dealing with temptation from people who are *intentionally* tempting you. These people either want you to fail, or they want you to succeed but are under the impression that enticing you with food is beneficial, that it will serve to "make you strong." The instant they discover that you are trying to control your eating, they make it their business to surround you with foods they know you should avoid.

The people who tempt you because they *want* you to fail are not always perceived as enemies. More often than not they are family members and friends. These people would never admit they are tempting you because they may not be consciously aware of it themselves. They may have a problem with envy or a low self-esteem. When this is the case, your success only serves to makes them feel worse about themselves, so they do things to make you fail.

The other type of intentional tempter has a mistaken idea that a constant exposure to whatever you find tempting will somehow strengthen your resistance. These are the people who think that surrounding you with foods that you should not eat will build up your immunity to desiring these foods in the same way our bodies do when they are exposed to germs. They don't understand the nature of temptation. Those things that are tempting are not like viruses and bacteria. We cannot "fight off" temptation the way we fight off the common cold.

Constant temptation does not make us strong—our appetite "immune system" is powerless to fight it, and we don't develop antibodies against the foods that entice us. To the contrary, on several occasions the apostle Paul instructs us to run the other way when we find ourselves faced with things that might lure us:

> Flee from sexual immorality.
> —1 CORINTHIANS 6:18

> Therefore, my dear friends, flee from idolatry.
> —1 CORINTHIANS 10:14

> But you, man of God, flee from all this [i.e., the love of money]...
> —1 TIMOTHY 6:11

Flee the evil desires of youth...
—2 TIMOTHY 2:22

According to Scripture, rather than expose ourselves to temptation, we should turn the other way, asking the Holy Spirit for the fruit of self-control to help us avoid those things that tempt us. We should also pray continually that the Lord guard us from things or people that have the potential to tempt us. Asking God in prayer to shield us from temptation not only makes common sense; it is also the way Jesus instructed us to pray. The Lord's Prayer, the familiar model prayer that Jesus gave His disciples, includes this request: "And lead us not into temptation, but deliver us from the evil one" (Matt. 6:13).

So what should you do with people who insist on tempting you? Sometimes you can't do anything other than hope they forget that you said you're trying to lose weight. But learn from the experience—use wisdom and discretion the next time before you speak. *Everyone* doesn't need to know your weight loss goals.

Tempted by ourselves

And finally, we are often the source of our own temptations. James 1:14 tells us that "each one is tempted when, by his own evil desire, he is dragged away and enticed." When we allow our minds to be preoccupied with thoughts about those foods that tempt us, we are setting ourselves up to be "dragged away and enticed."

The Holy Spirit gives us power to control *all* of our thoughts—even those thoughts that we find irresistible. Too many overweight and obese people spend too much time thinking about food. We should not let ourselves become preoccupied with what we'll eat, when we'll eat it, how we'll prepare it and what we'll serve it with.

Rather than dwell on things that ensnare us, the Bible tells us what things our minds should feast upon:

> Finally, brothers, whatever is true, whatever is noble, whatever is right, whatever is pure, whatever is lovely, whatever is admirable—if anything is excellent or praiseworthy—think about such things.
>
> —PHILIPPIANS 4:8

Biblical truths regarding temptation

Once we understand the various sources of temptation, we need to learn a few biblical truths regarding temptation. We have already looked briefly at Jesus' temptation in the wilderness. It is important that we grasp the significance of Jesus, our High Priest who intercedes to the Father on our behalf, being tempted: "Because he himself suffered when he was tempted, he is able to help those who are being tempted" (Heb. 2:18).

Jesus understands our pain. It is important to note that Jesus was tempted with food at a time when He hadn't eaten for forty days. He was genuinely hungry and had a real physical need for food. His situation is unlike ours many times when we yield to temptation in the absence of real hunger. A desire for the mere taste of the food (whether we're hungry or not) will cause many of us to yield to temptation.

Still, Jesus can relate to our struggle because He knows the pain of being seriously tempted with food. Who, then, is better equipped to intercede on our behalf than Jesus Christ? We should remind ourselves continuously that Christ is praying for us to be victorious in the face of temptation (Heb. 7:25).

Use the Word for your defense. Another thing worth noting about the manner in which Christ dealt with temptation is that He quoted the Word of God in His defense. Each time Satan came against Him, Jesus quoted Scripture. We cannot underestimate the importance of memorizing Bible verses, not only to handle temptation, but also as a source of encouragement, correction and strength. One passage that will be helpful for everyone trying to lose weight to memorize is 1 Corinthians 10:12–13:

> So, if you think you are standing firm, be careful that you don't fall! No temptation has seized you except what is common to man. And God is faithful; he will not let you be tempted beyond what you can bear. But when you are tempted, he will also provide a way out so that you can stand up under it.

This passage contains three key elements regarding temptation. First, it makes it clear that temptation is "common." Even though we don't all struggle in the same areas (for some, it's food; for others, it's pornography), we are all vulnerable to suffer temptation. In other words, we are not alone and our experiences are not isolated. Even during those times when we're convinced that no one alive could possibly be enticed *this* strongly by food, rest assured that there *is* someone who has felt exactly the same way as you do. We have not been singled out to struggle alone. Temptation is common; it is universal; everyone is tempted.

Sometimes just knowing this is sufficient to provide the extra surge of strength we need to overcome it.

The second thing this passage tells us is that even though temptation may seem to be unbearable, God has promised us that He will never allow us to suffer more than we can bear. The psalmist gave us a beautiful picture of how intimate our heavenly Father, who made us, knows and cares for us:

> O LORD, you have searched me
>   and you know me.
> You know when I sit and when I rise;
>   you perceive my thoughts from afar.
> You discern my going out and my lying down;
>   you are familiar with all my ways.
> Before a word is on my tongue
>   you know it completely, O LORD.
> You hem me in—behind and before;
>   you have laid your hand upon me...
>
> For you created my inmost being;
>   you knit me together in my
>   mother's womb...
> My frame was not hidden from you
>   when I was made in the secret place.
> When I was woven together in the depths of the
>   earth,
>   your eyes saw my unformed body.
> All the days ordained for me
>   were written in your book
>   before one of them came to be.
>   —PSALM 139:1–5, 13–16

God knows us better than we know ourselves. Most of us have no idea how much temptation we can bear because we yield long before we reach our limit. But when we feel like giving in, when we're at the brink of relinquishing self-control, we should remind ourselves that we *must* be equipped to resist this temptation because, as the apostle Paul wrote to the Corinthian church, our faithful Father "will not let you be tempted beyond what you can bear" (1 Cor. 10:13).

Once we have assured ourselves that God will not allow us to experience more than we can bear, then we proceed to the final truth from this passage of scripture—we look for the escape. Sometimes the means of escape is as simple as closing the refrigerator door and leaving the kitchen. It might require you to drive down a different street to avoid all your favorite fast-food restaurants. Whatever the case, instead of spending time struggling with the source of the temptation, immediately begin to look for what God has promised—a way out.

Learn to watch and pray. We should never lose sight of the fact that no matter how strong we think we are, we will always have the propensity to fall. Jesus warns believers to "watch and pray so that you will not fall into temptation. The spirit is willing, but the body is weak" (Matt. 26:41). Scripture warns us of our propensity to give in to temptation. They also promise us that though temptation is common, it won't be unbearable and we will be provided an escape route. (See 1 Corinthians 10:13.) In order to exercise self-control and resist temptation, we need to heed the words of Christ—watch and pray.

THE BENEFITS OF SELF-CONTROL

Along with protection from temptation and spiritual harm, the fruit of the Spirit of self-control also serves to enrich our lives.

Effective Christian lives

In the apostle Peter's second epistle, he discusses the benefits of adding godly virtues to our lives, including self-control:

> For this very reason, make every effort to add to your faith goodness; and to goodness, knowledge; and to knowledge, self-control; and to self-control, perseverance; and to perseverance, godliness; and to godliness, brotherly kindness; and to brotherly kindness, love. For if you possess these qualities in increasing measure, they will keep you from being ineffective and unproductive in your knowledge of our Lord Jesus Christ. But if anyone does not have them, he is nearsighted and blind, and has forgotten that he has been cleansed from his past sins.
> —2 PETER 1:5–9

These character traits make us productive and effective in our Christian lives. The converse is also true; when we lack self-control, for example, we set ourselves up for an ineffective and unproductive Christian life. A life that is rich in the knowledge of Christ is contingent upon our developing the fruit of self-control in our lives.

The apostle Peter continued in this passage to declare that when we lack these graces we become "nearsighted and blind" to spiritual and heavenly matters. We are blind to the redeeming power of Christ, whose shed blood gives us the strength we need to resist the temptations of the flesh, and we are nearsighted, focusing our attention on worldly desires rather than heavenly rewards.

When we yield to the lusts of the flesh, we not only hinder our personal growth, but we can also hinder the growth of the body of Christ. A church whose leadership is more concerned with "pleasing the masses" than confronting those members of the congregation who are actively engaged in the sins of the flesh is a weak church. Such a church is not equipped to make any significant contribution to building the kingdom of God.

Knowing the Lord our Healer

Another benefit that comes with practicing self-control is that we experience God as Jehovah Raphe, the Lord God our Healer. It is in the Book of Exodus where the Lord is revealed as our Healer:

> Then Moses cried out to the LORD, and the LORD showed him a piece of wood. He threw it into the water, and the water became sweet. There [at Marah] the LORD made a decree and a law for them, and there he tested them. He said, "If you listen carefully to the voice of the LORD your God and do what is right in his eyes, if you pay attention to his commands and keep all his decrees, I will not bring on you any of the diseases I brought on the Egyptians, for I am the LORD, who heals you."
>
> —EXODUS 15:25–26

What a wonderful reality: God *is* our healer. He has provided for our healing as described in His name: Jehovah Raphe. However, there are conditions surrounding this biblical promise of healing that we must accept as well as His promise to heal. This passage makes it clear that there were *conditions* that had to be met on the part of the Israelites in order for them to experience God as a healer. These conditions were the following:

- ✍ Listen carefully to the Lord.

- ✍ Do what was right in His eyes.

- ✍ Pay attention to His commands.

- ✍ Keep all His decrees (or statutes).

If they abided by these requirements, then God promised to spare them from experiencing the diseases He had brought on the Egyptians. If they failed to do so, then they could not rest in the assurance that God would manifest Himself as Jehovah Raphe and provide them with healing.

Some Bible scholars compare the land of Egypt to the world with all its bondage and sinful values. Our salvation through Christ is symbolized by the Israelites' deliverance from Egypt—we were once held in captivity as slaves to sin, but were miraculously redeemed through Christ, who freed us from the bondage of the world.

If Egypt symbolizes the world, what are some of the modern-day "diseases of the Egyptians"? They would be diseases that result from a disregard of the conditions set by God when He made the promise to be a healer. We have no assurance from the Lord that He will heal us from those diseases that result from committing the sin of idolatry or from yielding to the lusts of the flesh. These sins would place us in violation of the conditions that God established for healing.

Addiction—whether to tobacco, alcohol, drugs or food—is a form of idolatry. The addict yields allegiance to a *substance,* giving it authority to control his behavior. That authority belongs only to God. The substance, then, becomes an idol—something that is controlling and worshiped in the place of God. The Bible is clear that we should worship God alone.

Certainly committing idolatry would violate the conditions set by Jehovah Raphe. And we see evidence of this in the "diseases of Egypt" that plague us today. It is estimated that close to one million deaths per year are potentially preventable; they are the consequences of lifestyle choices. These diseases result from smoking (four hundred thousand tobacco-related deaths per year), drinking (one hundred thousand alcohol-related deaths per year), and overeating/inadequate activity (three hundred thousand diet- and exercise-related deaths per year).[1]

The fruit of the Spirit of self-control will help us to know God as our Healer by enabling us to adhere to the conditions required for healing. God *is* Jehovah Raphe, our Healer. And He has given us the Holy Spirit to equip us with the fruit of the Spirit. As we learn to yield to Him, we will enter into the benefits of healing as promised in the Scriptures.

FASTING AND PRAYER

Any Christian who is trying to lose weight must make fasting and prayer regular practices for life. Fasting and prayer keep us connected with God, the source of our strength. When we fast and pray, we maintain an intimate relationship with God. We have seen that He alone is the source of our strength, and He is the one who gives us power to cultivate the fruit of the Spirit, the divine secrets to living in victory over sin.

A commitment to fasting and prayer requires a tremendous amount of self-discipline and self-control. Giving these redemptive graces a high priority in our busy lives requires discipline; maintaining our focus during prayer and staying committed to a fast require self-control.

In the ninth chapter of the Gospel of Mark, we're given the account of Jesus' transfiguration. The latter part of this chapter tells us what happened when He and three of His disciples—Peter, James and John—came down from the mountain where He was transfigured. As they approached the crowds, an unidentified man knelt before Christ and asked that He heal his son. The man described the illness and added that Jesus' other disciples had tried, but they were unable to heal the boy. Jesus then healed the child in the presence of His disciples as well as a large crowd of scribes and onlookers.

Later, in a private meeting, His disciples asked Jesus why they were unsuccessful in bringing healing to the boy. Jesus responded, "This kind cannot be driven out by anything but prayer and fasting" (Mark 9:29, AMP).

Some problems can't be solved without tapping into the power of God through prayer and fasting. When we make these disciplines a regular part of our lives, God has promised that He will answer us and give us whatever we need to meet the challenges that face us.

Prayer accomplishes many things. It's a time to praise God; it's a time to ask God for wisdom and provisions; it's a time to thank God and a time to intercede on behalf of others. There is at least one other important purpose for prayer that cannot be overlooked: Prayer is a time to confess sin. The beloved disciple, John, wrote:

> If we claim to be without sin, we deceive ourselves and the truth is not in us. If we confess our sins, he is faithful and just and will forgive us our sins and purify us from all unrighteousness. If we claim we have not sinned, we make him out to be a liar and his word has no place in our lives.
> —1 JOHN 1:8–10

When we make the commitment to seek God's help in overcoming obesity, the first and crucial step is the confession of any sin that has contributed to the obesity, which may include the sins of idolatry and gluttony. According to Scripture, gluttony is a sin. It is included along with drunkenness in passages from Deuteronomy, Proverbs, Matthew and Luke. When we yield to the desires of our flesh by indulging ourselves with excessive amounts of food, we commit the sin of gluttony.

Gluttony, like sexual immorality, represents a perversion of a natural desire. It has become acceptable behavior because, unlike sex, which is *not* required to sustain our lives, eating *is* necessary for our survival. Consequently, the line that separates the normal act of "eating to live" from the gluttonous act of "living to eat" is readily crossed without much thought and without drawing much attention.

Gluttony is like the sin of sexual immorality in that there is "comfort in numbers." So many people fornicate and so many people overeat that we have become numb to the reality that these sinful behaviors grieve the Holy Spirit.

Gluttony is related closely to the sin of idolatry. Modern-day idolatry does not require us to bow down to statues and figurines as our ancient forefathers did. But as previously discussed, the sin of idolatry is committed when we worship the things that God has created and when we give them a control and authority in our lives that is reserved for God alone. Food fulfills this description.

Forgiveness for these sins of gluttony and idolatry require confession and repentance just like any other. As we humble ourselves to ask God to forgive us, He will, and we can begin to experience freedom from the bondage of that sin. The Holy Spirit longs to cleanse our temples and fill them with the glory of God manifested in the fruit of the Spirit we have discussed. These are the secrets to living in wonderful freedom from the bondage to sin and its consequences of obesity and being overweight.

Acknowledging sin

Our church is located in an area that has a high prevalence of drug addiction. In an effort to meet the needs of the community, we established a monthly deliverance service where we would pray for people specifically struggling with drug dependency. Those who attended regularly were the people who acknowledged their problem and knew they needed help from the Lord to overcome their addictions. They confessed that they were yielding to the desires of the flesh and had allowed themselves to be controlled by a substance rather than by God. Those addicts who refused to acknowledge that they had a problem, or those who were too proud to admit that they were powerless to overcome, usually stopped attending the services. They continued to use drugs and suffered the consequences of their addiction.

Over time, the deliverance service grew, and we found that the attendees were not only drug abusers, but also people who needed deliverance from other areas like smoking, pornography, alcohol and gambling. Overeaters, however, remained noticeably absent from these services. This reflects the prevailing attitude that indulging in food is not a sin, and, as such, it is not something that requires deliverance. This erroneous point of view is not unique to overeaters, but is common in our society. We are, in general, oblivious to the sin of gluttony.

I once told my husband that if our brothers and sisters struggling with alcoholism came into the congregation intoxicated, we would immediately pull them aside for correction and counseling. Depending on their degree of inebriation, we might even ask them to leave and return once they were sober. We have little tolerance for those who are addicted to mind-altering substances. Yet food addicts attend our services with little notice of their condition.

Most Christians have participated in services where a fellowship meal was served following the worship service. All too often, plates are piled high with enough food to feed several people. The guilty parties are not the poor or the homeless, who may not know when they'll have another decent meal, but Christians committing the sin of gluttony in the house of the Lord.

The passage from 1 John says that our purification comes with confession of sin. But it is rare to hear someone confess, "I eat too much." More commonly, there is defensiveness and denial of any wrongdoing. Unfortunately, when sin goes unconfessed, the behavior continues, and so do the consequences. In the case of gluttony, the consequences are severe: weight-related illnesses and premature death.

Repenting for our sin

After confession of sin comes repentance. Repentance means that we agree with God that our behavior is sinful, and then we choose to turn away from it. Fasting from food provides us the opportunity to draw closer to God and repent of anything that hinders our fellowship with Him. A spiritual fast is *not* a method for losing weight! We don't engage in a fast for the purpose of getting a boost in our weight-loss efforts. Just as praise dancing is not aerobic exercise, so spiritual fasting is not a way to jump-start a weight-loss plan.

A fast is a time to turn down the plate for the purpose of drawing closer to God. The minute you start to think about how many calories will be burned in the process, the focus is taken off God and placed on self. Your fast then becomes an exercise motivated by selfishness rather than a time of seeking God's face for meaningful fellowship. When spiritual acts are performed out of self-centeredness, they become useless rituals. Whatever is accomplished is minimal and insignificant.

In Matthew 6, Jesus teaches about fasting and prayer and mentions the religious hypocrites who fasted and prayed in order to draw attention to themselves and receive accolades from other less religious people. They did receive a reward: the recognition from those who were impressed by their "holiness." They missed the greater reward of recognition from God, who knew their hearts and knew their true motivation.

When a fast is motivated by personal gain, then the benefits will be small, just as they were for the hypocritical religious leaders. You will burn up a few hundred calories but miss the greater rewards of hearing from God, repenting from sin and growing stronger in faith and in the fruit of self-control. The calories burned in a selfishly motivated fast will re-accumulate after one visit to the ice cream parlor. But a fast done with the proper motivation will change your life.

Fasting is a practice that will facilitate our hearing from God as He reveals to us those things we need to change. Fasting then allows us to receive from God the power to implement the change. First comes repentance; then comes power.

Nehemiah is a wonderful Old Testament example of how powerful fasting and prayer can be. This faithful Jew was a cupbearer to King Artaxerxes I during the time that the Jews lived in exile in Persia. Some Jews had returned to Jerusalem, only to find the city and its surrounding walls (remember the importance of the walls) in a state of shambles. They reported this to Nehemiah:

> They said to me, "Those who survived the exile
> and are back in the province are in great trouble
> and disgrace. The wall of Jerusalem is broken
> down, and its gates have been burned with fire."
> When I heard these things, I sat down and wept.
> For some days I mourned and fasted and prayed
> before the God of heaven.
>
> —NEHEMIAH 1:3–4

Nehemiah's prayer is recorded in the verses following this passage. It is a prayer of confession and repentance for the sins the Israelites had committed that led to their captivity. Nehemiah demonstrates what true repentance is all about. When we fully appreciate how God perceives sin, we will mourn as Nehemiah did. Repentance is not a happy time; it is a time of deep sorrow. This is why sackcloth, a garment that symbolized humility and remorse, was commonly worn during the fast.

Christians have become so comfortable with the grace and mercy of God that we are prone to forget how offensive sinfulness is to Him. When we repent during a fast, our hunger and weakness can reinforce our feelings of contrition and remind us of how totally dependent we are on the very God that we've offended. And we know that He is faithful to forgive us of sin that we confess.

After Nehemiah confessed and repented, he received power and authority from God to do what he needed to do—rebuild the wall. He even received permission from a pagan king who was his captor to return to Jerusalem and to the work.

Rebuilding the wall was not an easy task. Nehemiah

faced a multitude of real and potential threats, and he had to overcome tremendous obstacles. But through it all, his dependency remained on God. Relying on the power of God for victory, Nehemiah succeeded because he never failed to recognize that he could do nothing without the help of the Lord:

> So the wall was completed on the twenty-fifth of Elul, in fifty-two days. When all our enemies heard about this, all the surrounding nations were afraid and lost their self-confidence, because they realized that this work had been done with the help of our God.
> —NEHEMIAH 6:15–16

This dramatic account of Nehemiah's victory demonstrates what can be accomplished through a spiritual fast. First comes repentance, and then comes power. When we sincerely repent of the sins of gluttony and idolatry, we can expect to receive the power we need to overcome them. This power is especially manifested in the fruit of the Spirit of self-control, though it is present in all the fruit of the Spirit.

For Nehemiah, having the power of God did not eliminate the need for discipline, perseverance and hard work. Likewise, tapping into the power of God and maturing in the area of self-control will not make losing weight an easy task but a possible one.

A patient once told me that her daily prayer was for God to completely remove her craving for sweets. I advised her not to hold her breath waiting. God has never promised to eliminate the many challenges of life. What He *has* promised is that He will never leave us or forsake us, and that He will be with us in trouble. He is our provider, our protector and the source of our strength. The psalmist eloquently describes these wonderful attributes of God:

> I lift up my eyes to the hills—
>   where does my help come from?
> My help comes from the LORD,
>   the Maker of Heaven and earth.
>
> He will not let your foot slip—
>   he who watches over you will not slumber;
> indeed, he who watches over Israel
>   will neither slumber nor sleep.
>
> The LORD watches over you—
>   the LORD is your shade at your right hand;
> the sun will not harm you by day,
>   nor the moon by night.
>
> The LORD will keep you from all harm—
>   he will watch over your life;
> the LORD will watch over your coming and going
>   both now and forevermore.
>
> —PSALM 121

This beautiful song was one of the Pilgrim Psalms, a collection of songs sung by those pilgrims traveling to Jerusalem for the annual feasts. What assurance and encouragement we have today, knowing that the God who proved to be a faithful *Keeper* to those ancient sojourners is the same God who will watch over us, guard us and be with us continually during our personal journeys of life. His presence is manifested within us in the person of the Holy Spirit, and the fruit of the Spirit equips us to be *more than conquerors* (Rom. 8:37) in all things and to experience a victorious—and healthy—life.

Enjoy the fruit!

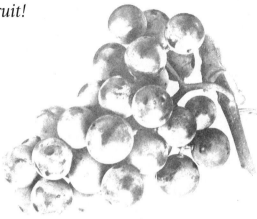

Afterword

Where there is no revelation, the people cast off restraint; but blessed is he who keeps the law.

—PROVERBS 29:18

This work was commissioned by God. I have attempted to the best of my ability to answer the Lord's call and write effectively what He has placed in my heart.

The incidence and prevalence of obesity has progressively increased over the past twenty years to the extent that it is now spreading with a rate that's similar to that of a communicable disease epidemic. Years ago, it became clear to me that this obesity epidemic has spiritual roots. But for whatever reason, the spiritual issues have gone unrecognized. The end result has been "superficial weeding"—we've plucked the dandelion at the base of the stem, but we've done nothing about the roots.

Our approach to the obesity epidemic has been superficial—we've tried diet plans, we've bought low-fat foods, and we've received prescriptions (and even operations) from our physicians—but we have failed to dig down and pull out the root for a permanent solution. Predictably, the problem hasn't gone away.

God has equipped us to go after the root. In the

apostle Peter's second letter, he tells the believers:

> His divine power has given us everything we need
> for life and godliness through our knowledge of
> him who called us by his own glory and goodness.
> Through these he has given us his very great and
> precious promises, so that through them you may
> participate in the divine nature and escape the
> corruption in the world caused by evil desires.
>   —2 PETER 1:3–4

Rather than use our power in Christ to "escape the corruption in the world caused by evil desires," we have done as the proverb indicates—we've "cast off restraint" when it comes to our eating and exercise habits. And now we are experiencing the consequences of excessive illness and premature death.

When the Lord showed me the spiritual nature of the problem, I felt a strong call to write it down and make it plain. I pray that this work has made a difference in your life and has served to remove any tendency to cast off restraints, and that it has instilled in you a stronger desire to abide by God's law. When this happens, prepare yourself to receive the blessing of better health.

—KARA E. DAVIS, M.D.

Appendix

Definition
of
Terms

Body Mass Index (BMI)—the current and preferred measurement for classifying body weight. Use the chart on pages 226–227 for determining your BMI.

Obesity—a BMI of 30 or more defines obesity. Obesity is further divided into three levels, obesity I, obesity II and extreme obesity III as indicated in the table on page 225.

Overweight—a BMI between 25.0 and 29.9 constitutes being overweight.

Weight-related illnesses—any of the illnesses that can be caused by, or exacerbated by, excessive body weight. These include type 2 diabetes mellitus, hypertension (high blood pressure), cardiovascular disease, high cholesterol, respiratory problems, sleep apnea, various cancers and osteoarthritis.

	OBESITY	BMI
Underweight		< 18.5
Normal		18.5–24.9
Overweight		25–29.9
Obesity	I	30–34.9
	II	35–39.9
Extreme Obesity	III	> 40

Body Mass Index Table

	Normal						Overweight					Obese					
BMI	19	20	21	22	23	24	25	26	27	28	29	30	31	32	33	34	35

Height (inches) — Body Weight (pounds)

Height	19	20	21	22	23	24	25	26	27	28	29	30	31	32	33	34	35
58	91	96	100	105	110	115	119	124	129	134	138	143	148	153	158	162	167
59	94	99	104	109	114	119	124	128	133	138	143	148	153	158	163	168	173
60	97	102	107	112	118	123	128	133	138	143	148	153	158	163	168	174	179
61	100	106	111	116	122	127	132	137	143	148	153	158	164	169	174	180	185
62	104	109	115	120	126	131	136	142	147	153	158	164	169	175	180	186	191
63	107	113	118	124	130	135	141	146	152	158	163	169	175	180	186	191	197
64	110	116	122	128	134	140	145	151	157	163	169	174	180	186	192	197	204
65	114	120	126	132	138	144	150	156	162	168	174	180	186	192	198	204	210
66	118	124	130	136	142	148	155	161	167	173	179	186	192	198	204	210	216
67	121	127	134	140	146	153	159	166	172	178	185	191	198	204	211	217	223
68	125	131	138	144	151	158	164	171	177	184	190	197	203	210	216	223	230
69	128	135	142	149	155	162	169	176	182	189	196	203	209	216	223	230	236
70	132	139	146	153	160	167	174	181	188	195	202	209	216	222	229	236	243
71	136	143	150	157	165	172	179	186	193	200	208	215	222	229	236	243	250
72	140	147	154	162	169	177	184	191	199	206	213	221	228	235	242	250	258
73	144	151	159	166	174	182	189	197	204	212	219	227	235	242	250	257	265
74	148	155	163	171	179	186	194	202	210	218	225	233	241	249	256	264	272
75	152	160	168	176	184	192	200	208	216	224	232	240	248	256	264	272	279
76	156	164	172	180	189	197	205	213	221	230	238	246	254	263	271	279	287

Source: Adapted from Clinical Guidelines on the Identification, Evaluation, and Treatment of Overweight and Obesity in Adults: The Evidence Report.

Body Mass Index Table

Obese						Extreme Obesity												
36	37	38	39	40	41	42	43	44	45	46	47	48	49	50	51	52	53	54

Height (inches)   **Body Weight (pounds)**

36	37	38	39	40	41	42	43	44	45	46	47	48	49	50	51	52	53	54
172	177	181	186	191	196	201	205	210	215	220	224	229	234	239	244	248	253	258
178	183	188	193	198	203	208	212	217	222	227	232	237	242	247	252	257	262	267
184	189	194	199	204	209	215	220	225	230	235	240	245	250	255	261	266	271	276
190	195	201	206	211	217	222	227	232	238	243	248	254	259	264	269	275	280	285
196	202	207	213	218	224	229	235	240	246	251	256	262	267	273	278	284	289	295
203	208	214	220	225	231	237	242	248	254	259	265	270	278	282	287	293	299	304
209	215	221	227	232	238	244	250	256	262	267	273	279	285	291	296	302	308	314
216	222	228	234	240	246	252	258	264	270	276	282	288	294	300	306	312	318	324
223	229	235	241	247	253	260	266	272	278	284	291	297	303	309	315	322	328	334
230	236	242	249	255	261	268	274	280	287	293	299	306	312	319	325	331	338	344
236	243	249	256	262	269	276	282	289	295	302	308	315	322	328	335	341	348	354
243	250	257	263	270	277	284	291	297	304	311	318	324	331	338	345	351	358	365
250	257	264	271	278	285	292	299	306	313	320	327	334	341	348	355	362	369	376
257	265	272	279	286	293	301	308	315	322	329	338	343	351	358	365	372	379	386
265	272	279	287	294	302	309	316	324	331	338	346	353	361	368	375	383	390	397
272	280	288	295	302	310	318	325	333	340	348	355	363	371	378	386	393	401	408
280	287	295	303	311	319	326	334	342	350	358	365	373	381	389	396	404	412	420
287	295	303	311	319	327	335	343	351	359	367	375	383	391	399	407	415	423	431
295	304	312	320	328	336	344	353	361	369	377	385	394	402	410	418	426	435	443

Source: Adapted from Clinical Guidelines on the Identification, Evaluation, and Treatment of Overweight and Obesity in Adults: The Evidence Report.

Notes

Introduction

1. A. H. Mokdad, M. H. Serdula, W. H. Dietz, B. A. Bowman, J. S. Marks and J. P. Koplan, "The Spread of the Obesity Epidemic in the United States, 1991-1998," *JAMA* 282 (1999): 1519–1522.

Chapter 1: The Fruit of the Spirit Is **Love...**

1. National Center for Health Statistics, *Third National Health and Nutrition Examination Survey*, 1988–1994.
2. W. S. Wolfe and C. C. Campbell, "Food pattern, diet quality, and related characteristics of school children in New York State," *J Am Diet Assoc.* 93 (1993): 1280–1284.
3. S. M. Krebs-Smith, A. Cook, A. F. Subar, L. Cleveland, J. Friday and L. L. Kahle, "Fruits and vegetable intakes of children and adolescents in the United States," *Arch Pediatr Adolescent Med.* 196; 150: 81–86.
4. "The painful business of losing weight," *The Economist* (August 30, 1997): 45–47.

Chapter 2: The Fruit of the Spirit Is **Joy...**

1. R. Schulz, S. R. Beach, D. G. Ives, L. M. Martire, A. A. Ariyo and W. J. Kop, "Association between depression and mortality in older adults: The Cardiovascular Health Study," *Arch Intern Med.*160 (2000) 1761–1768.
2. Z. N. Stowe and C. B. Nemeroff, "Women at risk for postpartum-onset major depression," *Am J Obstet Gynecol* 173 (1995): 639–645.
3. J. Unutzer, W. Katon, M. Sullivan and J. Miranda, "Treating depressed older adults in primary care: narrowing the gap between efficacy and effectiveness," *Milbank Q* 77 (1999): 225–256.
4. N. Frasure-Smith, F. Lesperance and M. Talajic, "Depression Following Myocardial Infarction: Impact on 6-month Survival," *JAMA* 270(15) (1993): 1819–1825.

5. P. A. Ades, "Cardiac rehabilitation in older coronary patients," *J Am Geriatr Soc* 47 (1999): 98–105.

6. W. Linden, C. Stossel and J. Maurice, "Psychosocial interventions for patients with coronary artery disease: a meta-analysis," *Arch Intern Med* 156 (1996): 745–752.

7. M. L. Fitzgibbon, M. R. Stolley and D. S. Kirschenbaum, "Obese people who seek treatment have different characteristics from those who do not seek treatment," *Health Psychol.* 12 (1993): 342–345.

8. B. T. Walsk, S. N. Seidman, R. Sysko and M. Gould, "Placebo Response in Studies of Major Depression: variable, substantial and growing," *JAMA* 287 (2002): 1840–1847.

Chapter 3: The Fruit of the Spirit Is *Peace...*

1. J. O. Prochaska, C. C. DiClemente and J. C. Norcross, "In Search of How People Change: Applications to Addictive Behaviors," *Am Psychol.* 47 (1992): 1102–1114.

Chapter 4: The Fruit of the Spirit Is *Patience...*

1. "Prevalence of overweight and obesity among adults: United States, 1999," *Health E-Stats* (Hyattsville, MD: National Center for Health Statistics, 2000).

2. F. X. Pi-Sunyer, "NHLBI Obesity Education Initiative Expert Panel on the Identification, Evaluation, and Treatment of Overweight and Obesity in Adults—the evidence report," *Obes Res* 6, supplement 2 (1998): 51S–209S.

3. S. L. Gortmaker, A. Must, J. M. Perrin, A. M. Sobol and W. H. Dietz, "Social and economic consequences of overweight in adolescence and young adulthood," *New England Journal of Medicine* 329 (1993): 1008–1012.

4. J. D. Sargent and D. G. Blanchflower, "Obesity and stature during adolescence and earnings in young

adulthood: analysis of a British birth cohort," *Arch Pediatr Adolesc Med* 148 (1994): 681–687.

5. P. Blumberg and L. P. Mellis, "Medical students' attitudes toward the obese and the morbidly obese," *Int Journal of Eating Disorders* 4 (1985): 169–175.

6. "He Looked Beyond My Fault" by Dottie Rambo. Copyright © 1968 John T. Benson Publishing Co. (ASCAP) (admin. by Brentwood-Benson Music Publishing, Inc.). All rights reserved. Used by permission.

Chapter 5: The Fruit of the Spirit Is **Kindness...**

1. Author unknown.
2. "Just a Closer Walk With Thee," anonymous. Public domain.

Chapter 6: The Fruit of the Spirit Is **Goodness...**

1. J. Salmeron, J. E. Manson, M. J. Stampfer, G. A. Colditz, A. L. Wing and W. C. Willett, "Dietary fiber, glycemic load and risk of non-insulin diabetes mellitus in women," *JAMA* 277 (1997): 472–477. J. Salmeron, A. Ascherio, E. B. Rimm et al., "Dietary fiber, glycemic load, and risk of NIDDM in men," *Diabetes Care* 20 (1997): 545–550.

2. M. Chandalia, A. Garg, D. Lutjohann, K. vonBergmann, S. Grunday and L. Brinkley, "Beneficial Effects of High Dietary Fiber Intake in Patients with Type 2 Diabetes Mellitus," *N Engl J Med* 342 (2000): 1392–1398.

Chapter 8: The Fruit of the Spirit Is **Gentleness...**

1. Agricultural Research Service, *Report of the Dietary Guidelines Advisory Committee on the Dietary Guidelines for Americans* (Washington, DC: Agricultural Research Service, 1995).

2. Institute of Medicine, *Weighing the Options: Criteria for*

Evaluating Weight Management Programs (Washington, DC: Institute of Medicine, 1995), 131.

3. *Diagnostic and Statistical Manual of Mental Disorders*, fourth edition (Washington, DC: American Psychiatric Association, 1994).

4. Source obtained from the Internet: "FDA announces withdrawal of fenfluramine and dexfenfluramine (September 15, 1997): www.fda.gov/cder/news/phen/fenphenpr81597.htm.

5. M. E. J. Lean, "Sibutramine: a review of clinical efficacy," *International Journal of Obesity* 21, supplement 1 (1997): S30–S36.

6. L. Sjostrom, A. Rissanen, T. Andersen et al., "Randomised placebo-controlled trial of orlistat for weight loss and prevention of weight regain in obese patients," *Lancet* 352 (1998): 167–172.

7. Source obtained from the Internet: "Number of liposuction procedures increase by 200 percent over five-year span" (Arlington Heights, IL: Plastic Surgery Information Service), available at www.plasticsurgery.org.

8. R. B. Rao, S. F. Ely and R. S. Hoffman, "Deaths Related to Liposuction," *N Engl J Med* 340 (1999): 1471–1475.

Chapter 9: The Fruit of the Spirit Is ***Self-Control...***

1. J. M. McGinnis and W. H. Foege, "Actual cases of death in the United States," *JAMA* 270 (1993): 2207.

For further information on the *Spiritual Secrets to Weight Loss*, you can contact Dr. Kara Davis at the following address:

Kara E. Davis, M.D.
P. O. Box 2491
Calumet City, IL 60409-9998

E-mail: KaraDavisMD@exgravedigger.com

You may also visit her website at:
www.exgravedigger.com

If you enjoyed *Spiritual Secrets of Weight Loss*, here are some other titles from Siloam Press that can help you to live in health—body, mind and spirit . . .

The Coming Cancer Cure
Francisco Contreras, M.D.
ISBN: 0-88419-846-4
Retail Price: $19.99

Dr. Francisco Contreras, a leading expert in cancer treatment, writes from a world platform of experience and recognition. He says, "We are beating cancer!" He outlines the latest findings in alternative cancer research and brings new testimonials from patients who have beaten the odds. Here families will find encouragement and a practical approach to the prevention and treatment of cancer.

Breaking the Grip of Dangerous Emotions
Janet Maccaro, Ph.D., C.N.C.
ISBN: 0-88419-749-2
Retail Price: $19.99

Learn how to stop letting dangerous emotions rob you of your joy as you discover the truth about worry and stress. You can replenish your physical body with a cutting-edge nutritional program that will restore your health. Explore exciting and proven protocols for rebuilding and regenerating your body, mind and spirit.

Walking in Divine Health
Don Colbert, M.D.
ISBN: 0-88419-626-7
Price: $10.99

Now you can know what foods have the potential to poison your body and what foods provide the greatest nutritional benefits for good health. Dr. Colbert thoroughly discusses the use of vitamins and minerals, giving many natural sources by which we can maintain our dietary needs for these substances.

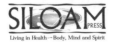

SILOAM PRESS
Living in Health—Body, Mind and Spirit

To pick up a copy of any of these titles, contact your local Christian bookstore or order online at www.siloampress.com.

Your Walk With God Can Be Even Deeper...

With *Charisma* magazine, you'll be informed and inspired by the features and stories about what the Holy Spirit is doing in the lives of believers today.

Each issue:

- Brings you exclusive world-wide reports to rejoice over.
- Keeps you informed on the latest news from a Christian perspective.
- Includes miracle-filled testimonies to build your faith.
- Gives you access to relevant teaching and exhortation from the most respected Christian leaders of our day.

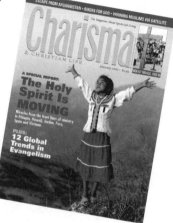

Call 1-800-829-3346 for 3 FREE trial issues
Offer #A2CCHB

If you like what you see, then pay the invoice of $22.97 (**saving over 51% off the cover price**) and receive 9 more issues (12 in all). Otherwise, write "cancel" on the invoice, return it, and owe nothing.

Experience the Power of Spirit-Led Living

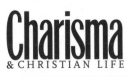

Charisma Offer #A2CCHB
P.O. Box 420234
Palm Coast, Florida 32142-0234
www.charismamag.com

1884A